Governing How We Care

Governing How We Care

*Contesting Community and Defining
Difference in U.S. Public Health Programs*

SUSAN J. SHAW

TEMPLE UNIVERSITY PRESS
Philadelphia

WITHDRAWN
UTSA LIBRARIES

TEMPLE UNIVERSITY PRESS
Philadelphia, Pennsylvania 19122
www.temple.edu/tempress

Library of Congress Cataloging-in-Publication Data

Shaw, Susan J., Dr.
  Governing how we care : contesting community and defining difference in U.S. public health programs / Susan J. Shaw.
      p. ; cm.
  Includes bibliographical references and index.
  ISBN 978-1-4399-0682-8 (cloth : alk. paper) — ISBN 978-1-4399-0683-5 (paper : alk. paper) — ISBN 978-1-4399-0684-2 (e-book)
  I. Title.
  [DNLM: 1. Public Health—United States. 2. Anthropology, Cultural—United States. 3. Community Health Services—United States. 4. Government Programs—United States. WA 100]

362.10973—dc23

2011040721

Printed in the United States of America

2 4 6 8 9 7 5 3 1

In memory of my father and in honor of my mother

Contents

Acknowledgments ix

Introduction 1

1 The Governmentality of Community Health 18

PART I Technologies of Citizenship and Difference

2 Community Health Advocates: The Professionalization
of "Like Helping Like" 43

3 Neoliberalism at Work: Contemporary Scenarios of
Governmental Reforms in Public Health and Social Work 72

4 Technologies of Culturally Appropriate Health Care 103

PART II Technologies of Prevention and Boundaries
of Citizenship: Drug Use, Research, and Public Health

5 "I Always Use Bleach": The Production and Circulation
of Risk and Norms in Drug Research 135

6 Syringe Exchange as a Practice of Governing 156

Conclusion 184

References 191

Index 211

Acknowledgments

I extend my sincere gratitude to the Wenner-Gren Foundation for Anthropological Research for its support of this work with the Hunt Postdoctoral Fellowship (2008–2009). Some of the research presented here was funded by the National Institute on Drug Abuse (R01 DA12569, Merrill Singer, Principal Investigator, and R03 DA16532, Susan Shaw, Principal Investigator), the Agency for Healthcare Research and Quality (R03 HS014086, Susan Shaw, Principal Investigator), the University of Arizona Social and Behavioral Sciences Research Institute's Faculty Summer Research Grant Development Stipend, and the University of North Carolina. I was fortunate to have the help and instrumental support of able research assistants, Julie Armin, Kathryn Orzech, Victor Reyes, and Tayana Richards. Julie Armin and Victor Reyes, in particular, contributed critical data analysis assistance to Chapter 4.

Thanks beyond words go to members of my various writing groups, which over the years have included Victor Braitberg, Thomas Chivens, Christopher Dole, Elizabeth Garland, Adam Geary, Thad Guldbrandsen, Stacey Langwick, Jennifer Roth-Gordon, Amy Stamm, and Terry Woronov. I literally would not have finished this project without their deadlines and thoughtful criticism. Sections of this book have been presented at the American Anthropology Association annual meetings; at the University of North Carolina, Department of Anthropology; at the University of California, San Francisco, Department of Anthropology, History and Social Medicine; and at the University of Arizona, Department of Gender and Women's Studies. I thank my colleagues in those settings, especially Laura Briggs, John Clarke, Adam Geary, Michele Rivkin-Fish, and Sandra Soto, for their helpful comments, which pushed me to clarify and strengthen my arguments. In addition, Michael Duke, Fletcher Linder, Lynn Morgan, Merrill Singer, Janelle Taylor, and anonymous reviewers for Temple University Press offered helpful insights and incisive critiques on chapters of the manuscript. An earlier version of Chapter 5 was previously published as Nancy Campbell and Susan Shaw, "Incitements to Discourse: Illicit Drugs, Harm Reduction and the Production of Ethnographic Subjects," *Cultural Anthropology* 23, no. 4 (2008): 688–717; I am grateful to my coauthor on that essay, Nancy Campbell, for moving my thinking on this material in productive directions. I have been fortunate to find a home for this book at Temple University Press, and I thank my editor, Mick Gusinde-Duffy, for his consistent support and encouragement throughout the process and the press for securing expert copyediting assistance.

My friends and colleagues at the place I call Thornton Community Health Center showed me every kind of hospitality, making Thornton a place I hated to leave. I remain indebted to them, and to our colleagues at the other Thornton organizations that supported my research, for their generosity; I regret any instance in which I have not lived up to their expectations. Friends in far-flung places have enlivened the seemingly endless process of writing with their ongoing interest and support, including Jessica Fields, Michael Hughes, Matthew King, Stacey Langwick, Diane Levy, Dale Morgan, Michelle Parrish, Carole Bowe Thompson, and Susan Weinrich. Every one of their gestures—reading drafts, making mix tapes, counseling me to continue—matters more than they can know. Members of my dissertation committee (Judith Farquhar, Sue Estroff, Dorothy Holland, and Della Pollock) set examples of intellectual achievement, each demonstrating unique ways of uniting theory and practice. I especially thank Judith Farquhar, mentor and role model, for her continuing interest in my work. My colleagues at the University of Arizona not only generously supported my time away to allow me to finish this book but also welcomed me to life in the desert with style and aplomb, for which I am grateful.

Finally, I thank my love and my partner in life, Amanda Quinby, for contributing the beautiful photographs that illustrate this book and for giving it, and me, more than I can say.

Introduction

Whehen I was an ethnographer for a federally funded study on HIV risk and needle use, I met Dave Wood, a middle-aged, slightly built African American heroin user who spent many of his days circulating through a neighborhood shopping plaza where people would arrive to get their morning coffee at McDonald's, pick up a loaf of bread at Sav-A-Lot, or buy and sell drugs in the parking lot. Dwayne Rogers, the outreach worker who was my partner on the study, introduced me to Wood. They had known each other for many years, starting from Rogers's own drug-using days when he spent time in that parking lot trying to hustle enough money for a fix. As a person in recovery and outreach worker for the project, Rogers served as a critical liaison between me and the people I was interested in recruiting as participants. In our first interview, Wood, like many people, worked hard to avoid being identified with a stigmatized group like injection drug users (IDUs), articulating a view of drug users that is clearly informed both by popular stereotypes and by the knowledge effects of the sort of research we were engaged in. Wood commented:

> See, you have different levels of people who use drugs. Like, . . . the guys I hang out with aren't the ones who are out on the street, the kind of people that you know, that you see always trying to scrape up ten dollars—you know, the kind of people you probably have interviewed, I should have put it that way. You know, you got people out there every day, they struggling

to survive and they look all greasy [*narrows his eyes*]. . . . People like that, they gotta be out there every day to get their twenty dollars for their drugs. See, I don't have to do that.

Wood's description of "the kind of people that [we] know" as state-funded ethnographers points to the complex processes involved in the production of difference through community health research. Wood's assertion that he was not among those who scrambled to get money to support a habit was particularly ironic, because over the course of many months I saw Wood engaged in exactly such activities in the Sav-A-Lot parking lot. One of his hustles might involve taking fifteen dollars from another user to buy her a bag of heroin for ten dollars and keeping five dollars as a "finder's fee," or he might do an in-depth interview with an ethnographer studying HIV risk in urban injection drug–using populations, receiving a twenty-dollar stipend for his participation. Wood's view of "the kind of people [we] know" and his effort to differentiate himself from them reveal more than the easily understood desire to distance oneself from an oft-disparaged group. His assertions also hint at the new subject-positions that are created for both researchers and participants as service delivery and disease surveillance converge in federally sponsored drug research.

Thornton,[1] where this fieldwork took place, is one of many deindustrialized New England towns and cities bypassed by the booming economy of the 1990s, whose fortunes have continued to decline since the departure of manufacturing jobs beginning in the 1970s. With the abandonment of the inner city, low-income and minority Thornton residents have experienced increasing poverty and health inequalities as indexed by an expanding HIV epidemic, especially among IDUs. African American and Latino community-based organizations have worked to politicize health inequalities such as disproportionate infant mortality or HIV rates in minority communities, drawing together diverse stakeholders under the banner of community health. This book tracks the history of several of these interventions to investigate community health as a key site in which public and scholarly ideas about racial and economic difference are elaborated. As advanced liberal government increasingly depends on the emergence and identification of populations as its mode of governing (Dean 1999), community health research plays a critical role in constituting those populations frequently deemed a "problem" for governing: the poor, minorities, and those who are socially or sexually marginalized. The case studies presented here show how community health research contributes

---

1. This is a pseudonym, as are all names of people, organizations, and places presented as part of the ethnographic data. I consider questions of anonymization at greater length later in this chapter.

to governance projects such as HIV prevention programs and shapes how people understand, participate in, and resist them.

In U.S. inner cities like the Thornton neighborhoods where this work is based, decisions about the health of the community have become a key if underrecognized battleground where state agencies try to manage unruly populations, and where members of marginalized groups stake claims for their health (see Biehl 2007). This book opens to analysis those bodies of knowledge that are produced and disseminated in decisions about how best to ensure the health and welfare of the community. Researchers and service providers in public health, social medicine, and primary health care have together produced the field of "community health," where minority and urban health issues are articulated in a context overdetermined by structural forces including deindustrialization, an expanding service economy, and increasing inequality. Further, neoliberal transformations in government displace responsibility for public health and welfare from public to private organizations. These developments have wide-ranging effects, including the constitution of new populations of "at-risk" or excluded citizen-subjects. Political theorist Nikolas Rose suggests, "[Neoliberalism] involves new conceptions of those who are to be governed, and of the proper relations between the governors and the governed. It puts new questions into play about the kinds of people we are, the kinds of problems we face, the kinds of relations of truth and power through which we are governed and through which we should govern ourselves" (Rose 1999, 188). Drawing on ethnographic research conducted between 1998 and 2004, this book places community health, a critically understudied area, at the center of analyses of contemporary transformations in governing.

As localities assume more and more responsibility for ensuring the public health, identity politics play an increasing yet largely unexamined role in public attitudes and policies. At the same time, the notion of "community" expands its previous meanings of territory and identity to become a central construct in governing (Creed 2006a). My analysis focuses not so much on the motives or understandings of individuals in government but rather on the disciplinary forms of knowledge and practice through which government is carried out—"the bodies of knowledge, belief, and opinion in which we are immersed" (Dean 1999, 16). In particular, I am concerned with the field of public health as an assemblage (Collier and Ong 2005) dedicated to the maintenance and promotion of a healthy population. Governing a healthy population takes place through a range of practices, including biomedical care, individual behaviors, and collective action. As a hybrid field combining elements of public health, medicine, and social medicine, community health brings to bear a special concern for the well-being of urban, poor, and minority populations. Community health research such as the HIV transmission study in which Dave Wood

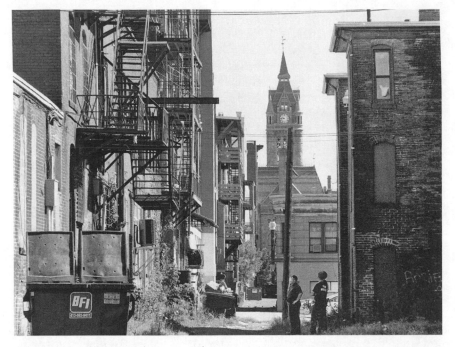

Alleys shelter injection drug users from prying eyes. *(Photograph courtesy of Amanda Quinby.)*

participated helps designate those marginalized populations, identities, and subject-positions occupied by their members.

Focusing on struggles over community health and health care in an age of neoliberalism, the three case studies presented in the two parts that follow examine the relationship between governing and the formation of politicized identities in the United States. Centered on the needs, demands, and concerns of the poor and marginalized, community health practitioners and researchers often find themselves engaged in highly politically and ethically charged activities, such as documenting the struggles of a woman addicted to heroin to locate a drug treatment program willing to accept her public health insurance as well as someone to care for her children while she detoxes. Struggles and debates over community health are shaped by larger contestations among individuals, organizations, and state actors over the meanings of cultural difference, morality, and justice. As groups lobby for more resources dedicated to African American health issues, for example, or debate the best way to prevent HIV in their communities, they take part in contestation over the art and practice of government.

This book presents a series of case studies—including a community health outreach program for women on welfare, online developments in culturally appropriate health care, and community debates over HIV prevention programs for IDUs—to analyze struggles around community health, governance, citizenship, and identity formation. In three related research projects conducted over six years, diverse actors make claims on the state as they strive to implement their visions of the social good and how the "conduct of conduct" (Foucault 1991) should be managed. Each study investigates the way that subject-positions are articulated through the structures, discourses, and practices of community health. I show practical examples of how community and cultural difference have come to function as new terrains of government, topographies that are traversed by variously positioned actors whose agendas often seem to head in different directions. This chapter briefly explores the political and epistemological challenges in conducting engaged, ethnographic community health research. I then outline how I came to be involved in each of the three projects, before giving an overview of the arguments presented in the chapters that follow.

The Politics of Ethnographic Knowledge and Practice

Activists must operate in an always uncomfortable space marked out on the one side by their will to bring about social justice and on the other side by their knowledge of their distance from those they support. —Andrew Metcalfe, "Living in a Clinic"

Ethical questions about the anthropologist's role, her relationships with her subjects, and shared social or political concerns are raised in particularly vivid terms by the experience of doing research in nonprofit settings, which often call for some form of pragmatic support or involvement by an ethnographer (Lyon-Callo 2004; D. Davis 2006; Hemment 2007). Research in impoverished settings in the United States frequently brings the ethnographer into contact with other disciplines such as health care, social work, or the law in ways that complicate the meaning of ethnographic fieldwork (O'Neil, Reading, and Leader 1998; Bourgois 1995). The possibility of ongoing working or personal relationships following fieldwork introduces opportunities for reciprocation and obligation in the ethnographer-subject relationship (Brettell 1993; Benjamin 1999; Weston 1991). For example, on the basis of participatory action research she undertook with a feminist group in Russia, Julie Hemment (2007) argues that ethnographic engagement not only deepens one's understanding of the exigencies that shape action but demands reflexivity as well. Like Hemment, I shared critiques of oppression and marginalization and goals of empowerment with the program staff I studied. In some instances this pushed me to take on more responsibility than was feasible, or effective.

Fieldwork is the practice of turning colors, chameleon-like, to suit one's environment, so the self that is extended bears only a certain resemblance to other selves that are performed in other parts of daily life. The critical junctures that arise from becoming vulnerable through interactions with others reveal in stark contrast the contradictions and occasional alliances between research goals, reciprocity, and obligation. Forming relationships with people with whom we do research implicates us in their goals and agendas. This was nowhere more evident than in the phrase Nikki Sparrow, my closest coworker at Thornton Community Health Center (TCHC) during my dissertation research, would use when she wanted my help with something: "Let me borrow your brain." John Caughey recommends, "I suggest that in studying any aspect of the culture we are personally involved in we should make explicit, systematic, rigorous use of our experiences" (1986, 242). I try to do the same here.

In her well-known essay "How Methodology Bleeds into Daily Life," Rayna Rapp observes that "working 'at home' has methodological, ethical, and interpretive consequences that would have been hard to foresee from the places I was initially trained to explore as an anthropologist" (1999, 16). Since then, our thoughts about what constitutes "home" have changed dramatically (B. Williams 1995; diLeonardo 2006) as the possible sites of home expand and as more and more anthropologists situate their work in the United States. Many politically engaged anthropologists (e.g., Lyon-Callo and Hyatt 2003) conduct ethnography in nonprofit and community-based organizations with which we share political, social, or economic goals.[2] We support the aims of such groups at the same time that they form our ethnographic subjects of study. As allies, and as ethnographers committed to the idea of "giving back," we commit our passion, time, energy, and expertise to supporting the aims such groups were established to meet, while remaining attentive to the unique epistemological privileges and costs of this engagement (Hemment 2007; Lassiter 2005).

I conducted most of the ethnographic fieldwork presented in these case studies in Thornton, a small New England rust-belt city whose population in the 2000 census was at least 21 percent African American and 27 percent Hispanic (predominantly Puerto Rican). In 1999, almost one-quarter of its residents lived below the federal poverty level. The burdens of poverty are not equally distributed, however: more than five times as many Latinos (42 percent) and three times as many African Americans (27 percent) as whites (8.2 percent) lived in poverty in 1999 (Harvard School of Public Health 2009). My research was concentrated in three neighborhoods that make up Thornton's "inner city." These neighborhoods—Williamsburg,

---

2. A large literature in anthropological methods and ethics proposes and critiques various engaged approaches to ethnographic research, including participatory, action, public, and radical anthropology (Polgar 1979; D. Davis 2006; Forman 1995; Lyon-Callo 2004; Singer 1993, 1994b). These and many other authors outline a diversity of ways to support the liberatory aims of people we study.

Brighton Square, and Nobb Hill—share high levels of unemployment, poverty, segregation, an expansion of the informal economy, and the retrenchment of public services, a combination of factors Allen Feldman (2001) terms "advanced marginality."[3]

The Williamsburg area is the historical center of Thornton's African American community, a tight-knit neighborhood that is home to a politically powerful African American middle class, several mosques, a sizable Caribbean population, and a small historic home district. In the early twentieth century, Brighton Square metamorphosed from an Italian American immigrant neighborhood to a working- to middle-class African American neighborhood. Many of these African American families were relocated in the 1960s when urban renewal brought freeways directly through their previously prosperous neighborhood. As part of this demographic transition, more recently arrived Puerto Ricans from New York, New Haven, or other, poorer sections of Thornton moved into the vacated housing, taking advantage of cheap rents and higher-quality housing stock. In contrast to Nobb Hill's very transient Puerto Rican population, Latinos in Brighton Square remained and built a number of stable and successful community organizations.

Nobb Hill, a neighborhood completing its conversion from Italian American to Puerto Rican residents, is home to TCHC, a federally funded clinic that sponsored the Community Health Advocate (CHA) program discussed in Chapters 2 and 3. The patient population at TCHC was nearly evenly divided among African Americans, Latinos (over 85 percent of whom were Puerto Rican), and Russian and Vietnamese immigrants at the time of my research. The health center offered bilingual practitioners and a full complement of medical translators. All signs in the health center were posted in at least four languages: English, Spanish, Russian, and Vietnamese. A disproportionately large (relative to population) percentage of patients were Russian and Vietnamese because Thornton was a refugee resettlement area and TCHC had a contract with the state to provide refugee health assessments.

I came to Thornton beginning in 1998, when I was searching for a site for my dissertation fieldwork. I was choosing between two very different community health centers. Both were located in small Massachusetts cities that exemplified conditions of advanced marginalization, but one clinic was decades old while the other, TCHC, was more recently established. One site was ethnically homogenous, while the other served a diverse immigrant population. I was intrigued by the possibilities and challenges inherent in the concept of developing a health center "by and for the community" when "the community" was made up of so many diverse groups,

---

3. As explored in Part II, these neighborhoods also share a strong association in the local media with drug use, HIV, and minority populations.

and I chose to study TCHC. Because the CHA program, the subject of Chapters 2 and 3, was just getting underway at the time I started my fieldwork, the executive director suggested that I take that program as my particular focus (though he granted me full access to all parts of the clinic except doctor-patient clinical encounters).

Without its own building throughout the duration of my fieldwork, TCHC occupies a series of rented spaces in the Nobb Hill section of Thornton. The clinic is a warren of low-slung, single-story offices on a street that seems to be continually undergoing redevelopment. Administrative; Women, Infants, and Children (WIC); and outreach staff work across the street in an office building that also houses many attorneys-at-law. The pragmatic and symbolic divide between these functions of the organization represented by the busy main street of Thornton loomed large throughout my fieldwork. Clinical staff typically did not socialize with administrative, WIC, or outreach staff, who generally did not understand the work performed by their colleagues across the street. Especially at the beginning of my fieldwork, many habits and systems of work at the clinic were in the process of being developed, and the gaps and affiliations illustrated by this spatial divide proved significant for years to come.

Questions of reciprocity and obligation became increasingly salient as my dissertation fieldwork progressed. Over time my participant-observation research became more and more participatory as I began to assume some of the responsibilities of coordinating the CHA program. I was torn between the desire to provide pragmatic help and the desire to maintain my freedom and some semblance of distance. When the health promotion unit head, Nikki Sparrow, asked me if I would be willing to work for the health center as the part-time coordinator for the CHA program, I realized where my boundaries lay in terms of involvement. While I may have been taking on some parts of the job, to be an actual staff person at the health center would have represented a significant change in my role. Being directly and personally implicated in TCHC's structures of accountability would have dramatically altered my relationships with the lead health educator, health advocates, and other program coordinators, a change I ultimately could not accept. Despite this decision, however, as time passed my field notes increasingly began to open with to-do lists, and "things to do" would crowd the margins. I took on prosaic responsibilities such as providing transportation for CHAs to distant, off-site training. I saw these tasks as opportunities for spending time with participants in different venues—but once I committed to help, it became a responsibility all the same.

In an effort to protect research participants from further public scrutiny, ethnographers often work to conceal the identities and even the locations of the people we write about (Brettell 1993; Apter et al. 2009; A. Stein 2010). When we discussed the politics and possibilities of anonymity for

TCHC in any published work that might result from my research, TCHC's executive director at the time I began my dissertation fieldwork confidently assured me that I was welcome to name the organization, perhaps because he imagined this would lead to greater recognition for its achievements. Despite this, I have elected to change the names of all individuals, organizations, and locations in keeping with anthropological convention. However, unique features of Massachusetts law shaped the parameters of my fieldwork and must therefore be included here. Massachusetts state laws prefigured later federal developments on at least two occasions that are relevant to this story. Massachusetts passed a version of welfare reform several years before the 1996 federal welfare reform law was passed. In contrast, Massachusetts was an anomaly in HIV prevention policy for many years, remaining one of only a handful of states that prohibited the sale of syringes over the counter until 2006. Further, a critical element of the story told in Chapter 6 concerns the Massachusetts law requiring syringe exchange programs (SEPs) to obtain "local approval," pushing responsibility onto localities as a means of protecting state legislators from the wrath of syringe exchange opponents. I proceed with this strategy of anonymization with some uncertainty but with the hope that it offers the best solution to the need to account for relevant context while respecting the privacy of people and organizations who shared their professional and personal lives with me.

"Empowering" Community Health Advocates

The CHA program discussed in Part II was developed as a form of "radical health education" (Minkler 1992; Minkler and Wallerstein 1997) to foster greater self-determination among those who are the "targets" of health and social programs (Gastaldo 1997). Similar to the aims of some activist anthropologists (Lyon-Callo 2004), radical health education seeks to overturn what they see as the oppressive power relations inherent in traditional research in favor of a more committed, cooperative, and participatory approach to public health and research (see, e.g., Harrison 1991; Park 1993; Polgar 1979). Likewise, the cultural competency proponents presented in Chapter 4 see themselves as activists in the movement to bring social justice and antiracist education to the field of health care.

I shared many of the goals of the CHA program designers, Mercedes Cota and Niara Kadar, two community health organizers who together facilitated the six-week-long participatory training for new CHAs. They sought to provide resources for low-income African American and Latina women to become agents of change for their communities, using health disparities as the fulcrum with which to mobilize others. Especially at the beginning of my fieldwork, I supported both the aims and the model of the CHA program, which made it even easier to become fully immersed in its nuts-and-bolts operations. I tried to imagine how my ongoing fieldwork could be used to support the program and advance its aims. Implementing the CHA program brought a plethora of difficulties once the health advocates completed their training and started work at their respective agencies, however, as Viviana's experiences illustrate.

While many women whom we tried to recruit for the program wanted nothing more than regular, middle-class, or professional jobs that paid them a living wage so they could provide for their families, others seemed excited by the opportunity to be a CHA. For many, it was their first chance to relate to others in a supportive pedagogical environment. For instance, on the second or third day of the training, I overheard Viviana repeating to herself, "I love this. I love this," as she sat next to me. Viviana was the only Puerto Rican participant in our class of about twenty African American and Caribbean American participants. As a fully bilingual Spanish speaker, she was a valuable asset to the outreach team for TCHC who would be working in predominantly Puerto Rican neighborhoods. I got to know her well on the thirty-minute drive to and from the training each day. As outsiders together we formed a kind of alliance in the training, either sitting next to each other or else grouped together by other participants. In some ways Viviana relished her difference from the others, expounding at length on Puerto Rican culture and traditions. At other times she asserted a shared identity with other participants as people of color, saying, "I'm Spanish, but I'm black inside." Her efforts in establishing this kind of solidarity were met with bemused acceptance by African American participants. Everyone agreed on her nickname, "the Mayor," because she greeted everybody by name and with a handshake daily. Viviana's early penchant for this kind of participation led to her eventual departure from the program for a better job, because the health center was too disorganized to give her satisfying work and because—since she was no longer a welfare recipient—the part-time work did not pay her a living wage.

At TCHC, Viviana was among the most vocal critics of the health center's failure to provide appropriate accommodations for the CHAs. While she often helped try to smooth over the grumblings of other participants, her eventual defection for a secretarial job in the housing office of her Section 8 building marked both a success of the program (in moving a former welfare recipient into stable, full-time work) and its failure to accommodate and build on Viviana's genuine efforts to help others. She showed a flair for the role of advocate as she accosted people on the street and helped them negotiate the bureaucracies of Medicaid, and I was almost as disappointed as she was by our failure to keep her. Programs such as the CHA program do have an obligation to the people they recruit, an obligation to leave them better off, in some way, than when they began—and yet so many programs (and researchers) fail to meet these obligations, for many reasons.[4] Funding for the CHA program ended, some CHAs were hired into other positions at TCHC, and the clinic itself entered a phase of fiscal crisis accompanied by widespread layoffs and reorganization. I still ponder how or whether the research presented here was able to forward the CHA program's aims, though my next two Thornton research studies, focused on HIV risk among IDUs, provided more concrete ways to contribute to policy debates that emerged around community health programs. Concurrently, however, I continued another small research project focused on culturally appropriate health care.

Producing and Addressing Differences in the Clinic

The production, reproduction, and dissemination of new formulations of ethnic and racial identities through discussions in the clinic about how to provide more culturally appropriate health care drove me to seek out other domains in which ethnic and cultural difference is produced in medical encounters. Online efforts to develop culturally appropriate health care respond to the same problems of *difference* and *distance* addressed by the lay health outreach worker program presented in Chapters 2 and 3. I was introduced to the Culture and Health e-mail discussion list, which forms the basis of material analyzed in Chapter 4, when a colleague forwarded me a message from the list. The Culture and Health list unites participants from all over the world to disseminate marginalized forms of expertise that have been mobilized as ethical-political solutions to the "problem" of cultural difference in health care. A moderator screens messages and posts them to the list and subscribes individuals. Reflecting expanding interest in topics of culture and health across public health and the health professions, the number of subscribers to Culture and Health has grown steadily; when I first subscribed in 2003, the list reached about two hundred members, while in 2007 the moderator announced that she had signed up the one thousandth list member, and in 2010 that number was nearing two thousand subscribers. Those who post to the list tend to be health care administrators who have been assigned responsibility for handling issues related to "cultural diversity," such as medical interpreters, or for ensuring compliance with federal regulations. A few nursing academics, medical anthropologists, and cultural competence "experts" who seek to share expertise and market their services also post regularly. I also explored the

---

4. In *The Will to Improve*, Tanya Li outlines the often-unintended consequences of improvement programs carried out in colonial and postcolonial circumstances (Li 2007), including the seeding of new "problems" that later serve as justifications for further improvement programs. Kate Crehan (2006) points out the broad similarities between the language used in domestic U.S. urban redevelopment and international development literatures. These broad patterns are explored further in Part I, particularly around themes of empowerment, responsibility, and participation.

online training modules and curricula through which "cultural expertise" is transmitted and shared from trainers and administrators to health care providers themselves. The first time I presented this work as a lecture, audience members urged me to seek out sites where cultural competence trainers, administrators, and other health care workers meet in person, to supplement my analysis of the online posts with observations of face-to-face encounters. So I attended several conferences and training sessions devoted to topics related to culturally appropriate health care.

Around this time, I was invited to contribute a guest lecture on cultural competence to an online gerontology course on health literacy. I hesitated—since much of my work on cultural competence had involved critiquing the oversimplifications and subject-producing effects of cultural competence discourse and interventions, I was not sure it made sense to be actively involved in producing and disseminating such knowledge, even in a seemingly innocuous setting like this. When I discussed the invitation with my partner, she pointed out that this would provide another opportunity for participant-observation research and that I might be able to learn more by taking part in the production and circulation of cultural competence knowledge.

I created PowerPoint slides and a digital audio recording of a lecture that outlined anthropological understandings of culture and explanatory models of illness (including biomedical explanatory models) and presented overviews of several approaches to cultural competence (see Chapter 4). Students were required to write brief essays responding to the assigned readings and my lecture and, in a subsequent online discussion, to apply concepts from the lecture or readings to their own experiences as either employees or students. Many students were enrolled a pharmacy program, bringing several years' experience working as pharmacy techs in retail pharmacies in Tucson and elsewhere. Their online comments about these experiences etched in sharp relief the inequalities of access that drive cultural competence educators to redouble their efforts. Students described trying to communicate across language gaps using "hand gestures," "facial expressions," and "hoping for the best." Impromptu interpreters that students reported recruiting to help them communicate with their customers included "an employee who may be working in the cosmetics department," other customers, or a patient's son or daughter. While members of the Culture and Health list and participants in cultural competence conferences often use similar stories of gaps in care to ground their claims for cultural competence interventions, these vivid cases of substandard access to medication information related by students (who thought they were doing an adequate job of delivering care) nonetheless shocked me, illustrating yet again what poor care passes as sufficient for linguistic minorities in the United States.

Putting together a forty-five-minute lecture, delivered online to students I would never meet, did help me appreciate the frustration that cultural competence trainers frequently vent on the Culture and Health list about the challenge of reducing complex concepts such as cultural difference to sound bites delivered with the intention of improving care. I was concerned about the oversimplifications I presented in my lecture, and yet, as became clearer to me only after the task was completed, the problems I sought to address are real.[5] This tension between the inadequacy of remedies (which are themselves plagued by a raft of unintended consequences) and the profound gaps in quality of health care for the poor and marginalized animates all the case studies discussed here.

Illicit Drug Use, HIV Prevention, and Marginalization

I returned to Thornton after an absence of about three years as an ethnographer with the Hispanic Health Council in Hartford, Connecticut. Resuming fieldwork in Thornton, as part of a three-city study on HIV risk and injection drug use, I was dismayed to discover that little had changed during my absence. The "roaring Nineties" seemed to have bypassed the city altogether. Abortive redevelopment projects would occasionally install new facades on downtown music venues or restaurants, but a year later the spaces usually stood empty. TCHC struggled with declining Medicaid reimbursements and changes associated with Massachusetts's own welfare reform and health insurance reform laws (which eliminated the state's "Free Care" pool, which safety-net health care providers used to reimburse themselves for care they provided to the uninsured). The clinic teetered between the brink of disaster and winning accolades for its innovative health promotion work conducted on shoestring budgets by dedicated staff members. Staff turnover continued apace, such that ten years later almost none of the original staff members I met during my dissertation fieldwork are still employed there.

Between 2001 and 2003 I worked as an ethnographer based at Thornton Community Health Center and at the Brighton Square Community Health Coalition (a group of health care and other service providers that was also active in the CHA program), where I worked closely with two outreach workers. Though employed by the Hispanic Health Council, I was the Thornton site ethnographer for the Syringe Access project, a study of syringe-related HIV risk funded by the National Institutes of Health. Ethnographers and outreach workers for the Syringe Access study were also

---

5. As a development worker said to ethnographer Tanya Li after she outlined her critique of development programs in Indonesia, "You may be right, but we still have to do something. We can't just give up" (Li 2007, 2).

based in each of the two Connecticut research sites, with support and coordination provided by the Hispanic Health Council and investigators at Yale University and the University of Massachusetts. Much of the ethnography presented in Chapter 5 was completed with the support of that project.[6]

As an ethnographer for a study of HIV risk among IDUs, I became better acquainted with the fragile, tenuous connection between primary health care and behavioral and mental health resources for the poor and underserved. Public debates on drug use and HIV, which reached a fever pitch during my 1998 fieldwork with the citywide referendum that defeated syringe exchange, continued as public health advocates pressed for prevention programs while opponents dug in and marshaled their objections (Shaw 2006). AIDS activists had struggled for years to open an SEP to prevent HIV among IDUs in Thornton, where 52 percent of new AIDS cases were attributable to injection drug use in 2001 (MDPH 2001). SEP advocates failed to mobilize the active support of African American voters, many of whom see substance abuse (and HIV infection) as an important index of their community's marginalization (Shaw 2006).

To learn more about why such diverse groups opposed syringe exchange so vehemently, I developed a small study of community attitudes toward syringe exchange, drawing on both household survey and ethnographic methods.[7] With a team of community interviewers, my collaborators and I completed door-to-door surveys in English and Spanish. I also conducted participant-observation research with syringe exchange organizations in Connecticut, which faced their own budget cuts, local opposition, and other organizational challenges.

I was invited to present findings from this research in public hearings at both the local and state level. Most of the African American and Latino residents we interviewed supported syringe exchange to prevent HIV infection, while opponents were more likely to be white and suburban. This data also supported arguments for neighborhood-based representation on the Thornton City Council instead of the at-large system used for forty years, since the white-majority city council had repeatedly opposed syringe exchange while most residents of Thornton's inner city favored it (see Chapter 6). Research I conducted with harm reduction programs portrayed in Chapters 5 and 6 was based both in Thornton and at several area SEPs, and it continued throughout both the Syringe Access project and the Community Attitudes study. My interviews for that study were completed between 2001 and 2005 with IDUs in Thornton's three "inner city" neighborhoods, as well as with staff from area SEPs.

6. The project was funded by the National Institute on Drug Abuse (R01 DA12569, Merrill Singer, Principal Investigator).

7. The study was funded by the National Institute on Drug Abuse (R03 DA16532, Susan Shaw, Principal Investigator).

Project Overview

This book unites theoretical analyses of the relationship between government and citizens with clinic-based and community studies of on-the-ground struggles over the meaning of cultural difference, ethnicity, and belonging among diverse communities in urban Thornton, Massachusetts. Chapter 1 provides a theoretical overview of the major concepts that run throughout the book. Part I, "Technologies of Citizenship and Difference" (Chapters 2 to 4), explores a range of social, practical, and electronic technologies that mediate subjects' relationships with health care organizations and the state, including the CHA program, which trained low-income women of color to serve as public health outreach workers, and the emergence of cultural competency programs as ethical-political solutions to the "problem" of cultural difference in health care. CHAs were to serve as bridges between underserved communities and the community health agencies that employed them, engaging residents in a process of community empowerment. Women on welfare who enrolled in this program began a course of self-fashioning that started with participatory education for "empowerment" and closed with the habits and skills necessary for the "world of work" when the program began to receive federal Welfare-to-Work (WtW) funding midway through my fieldwork. Chapter 2, "Community Health Advocates: The Professionalization of 'Like Helping Like,'" describes a Freirean training for low-income women of color to serve as outreach workers in underserved neighborhoods. I trace the ways in which "community" was mobilized throughout this program and produced as a sign with meanings of nonprofessional authenticity (similar to street credibility), ethnic identity, and contradictory implications of marginalization and belonging. In the CHA program, notions of community are linked to ethnicity through technical and administrative practices, as well as through community organizing efforts that function as practices of identity.

Chapter 3, "Neoliberalism at Work: Contemporary Scenarios of Governmental Reforms in Public Health and Social Work," outlines the transformations that the CHA program underwent when it received WtW funding to support CHA salaries. Aimed at creating productive citizens, Massachusetts's welfare reform law specified a new population, the "hardest to serve," and sought to use community empowerment to move them from dependency to self-sufficiency. The WtW program instituted new governing relationships and disciplinary practices that were designed to transform welfare recipients. Participation in the WtW program made Thornton Community Health Center and its partner agencies subject to the discipline of the state in new ways as well.

These themes of the management of difference through community health are also addressed in the second case study in Part I. Chapter 4,

"Technologies of Culturally Appropriate Health Care," explores the development and dissemination of cultural expertise to health professionals through online media, drawing on five years of contributions to an e-mail discussion list on culturally appropriate health care and on participant-observation research at conferences and trainings. As minority advocacy groups and others seek to make health care more inclusive, new interventions are being developed to reform health care and expand the regimes of knowledge that are available to health care providers. An emerging "cultural competence" industry generates and distributes specialized social expertise using online media to teach health care providers how best to respond to "cultural difference" in clinical encounters. In many public health and primary care settings, outreach workers are used to reach those whose cultural difference is assumed to keep them *out* of the clinic (making them "hard to serve"), while trainings for physicians are meant to help them deal more effectively with cultural differences in clinical encounters. Both types of programs have the simultaneous effect of *producing* new understandings of difference as they strive to negotiate and resolve it. Further, culturally appropriate health care aims to eliminate health disparities by governing the conduct of both medical professionals and patients.

Part II of the book, "Technologies of Prevention and Boundaries of Citizenship: Drug Use, Research, and Public Health," explores another dimension of community health: that focused on substance abuse and HIV prevention. Part II features ethnographic research I conducted between 2001 and 2004 with injection drug users (IDUs) to investigate the intersections among community health research and the formation of identities and populations. Chapter 5, "'I Always Use Bleach': The Production and Circulation of Risk and Norms in Drug Research," traces the circulation of "harm reduction" discourse through researchers' interactions with drug users. Harm reduction is a pragmatic approach designed by drug users themselves aimed at reducing the negative health and social effects of drug use through modest interventions in drug use behaviors (Marlatt 1996). In the wake of the HIV/AIDS epidemic, harm reduction activists focused on reducing the risk of HIV transmission through contaminated injection equipment. Their practices and pedagogy were influenced by findings from sympathetic drug researchers whose work helped shape new norms of drug-using behavior. Carrying out state-funded drug ethnographies places researchers in the position of *representing* to IDUs these principles of HIV risk reduction (for example, "don't share syringes"), in relation to which drug users locate their own practices to establish themselves as ethical subjects if not citizens.

In Thornton, AIDS activists have struggled for years without success to open a SEP to prevent HIV among IDUs. Syringe exchange, explored in Chapter 6, "Syringe Exchange as a Practice of Governing," is a hotly contested practice that enacts both the state's and the public's ambivalent relationship with drug use and drug users. Harm reduction practices, like other public health and primary care programs, work to manage populations by serving them through a range of specific accounting practices. Organizations rely on a variety of techniques, from tagged syringes to one-for-one exchanges to mass distribution programs, to regulate the circulation of and access to syringes with a range of effects on staff, users, and public perceptions of the role and purpose of syringe exchange as a technology for HIV prevention.

As with other terrains of social life such as welfare and sexuality, community health is implicated in questions of government in complex ways. Public health institutions seek to redistribute health care and mobilize other techniques of government that engage individual citizens by weaving together concepts of identity and difference into the notion of "community" as a terrain of government. As communities mobilize health statistics to support their political arguments and demands, however, their voices are being articulated in a political environment that is increasingly governed by neoliberal thought—an environment whose dominant rationality relies on the logic of a competitive marketplace in addition to, or perhaps even instead of, claims of justice.

1

The Governmentality
of Community Health

Governmentality, as defined first by Michel Foucault (1991) and elaborated by subsequent social theorists and anthropologists (e.g., Inda 2005; Ong and Collier 2005), explores the knowledge formations and sets of practices that together work to construct and govern populations and subjects. Drawing on the case studies that follow, I contend that community health practices represent a privileged site for examining the "conduct of conduct"—the norms, etiquette, and behavior of individuals and populations—because the populations targeted by community health interventions are constituted, in part, by their difference. As health care and prevention are increasingly imbricated in a wide range of social practices (Briggs 2003), and as the United States undergoes yet another paroxysm of health care reform, community health research and practice are becoming key arenas in which new forms of subjects are produced. This book explores state and nonstate actions designed to "ethicalize" health care (Rose 1998, 91) by expanding access to health care, addressing cultural difference in the clinic, and preventing HIV among people who use injection drugs.

To carry out this analysis, we must first consider how health policy and practice, including community organizing around health issues, can be a site for the production of subjects. This chapter discusses the diverse meanings of ethnicity and community that contribute to the formation of the field "community health," including constructions of ethnicity as a category of governing. This work extends the anthropological concept of biosociality (Rabinow 1996) to understand the ways in which marginalized groups mobilize, using health issues as a fulcrum and inequality as the lever to shift structures and their alignments that lead to their immiseration. In the chapters that follow, we see a range of community groups present health disparities arguments as a key means of circulating and disseminating claims for resources and recognition. This chapter discusses the main theoretical concepts that run through all three case studies.

Research and health promotion practices enable the government of citizen-subjects, forming new subject-positions such as the public health outreach worker and the ethical drug user (Campbell and Shaw 2008). Questions of everyday practice make up the heart of the material under investigation here, as I shift the lens of biosociality from people's interactions with the knowledge and technologies of biomedicine to the city street, where those with less access to health care contest their exclusion using the language of health disparities. Community activists, including public health workers and former drug users, establish organizations and programs designed to improve health access as a means of instantiating the very communities such programs hope to serve (Crehan 2006). In tracing these developments, I follow the direction pointed out by Nikolas Rose in *Powers of Freedom* (1999). A "historian of the present" regards current social configurations as "an array of problems and questions, an actuality to be acted upon and within by genealogical investigation" (1999, 11). The historian of the present examines those "configurations of the minor" (1999, 31)—the small changes in drug users' behavior, for example, recommended by the U.S. Centers for Disease Control and fostered by harm reduction programs to limit HIV infection—which illuminate broader social trends such as the increasing emphasis on individual responsibility for health and prevention. By tracing the networks in which actors (agencies, health care providers, neighborhoods) act, examining the resources they use, and identifying the circumstances that shape their actions, this book offers an empirical examination of the social and economic changes taking place in the way government happens.

Community Health and the Production of Difference

In anthropology, history, and social theory, a wide body of scholarship has described the clinic as a site for the production of subjectivity (e.g., Foucault 1975, 1991; Kleinman 1980, 1988; Scheper-Hughes and Lock 1987, among many others). Medical expertise combines with state power and authority to create categories that subjects come to inhabit, such as "person with AIDS," breast cancer survivor, or homosexual (Foucault 1978; Glick Schiller, Crystal, and Lewellen 1994; Treichler 1989; Klawiter 2008; Lorway, Reza-Paul, and Pasha 2009). However, far less has been written on the production of ethnicity in the clinic. In their book *Ethnicity,*

Inc., anthropologists John and Jean Comaroff outline three recent factors that contribute to the increased visibility of "the presence of 'others' within" the nation-state (Comaroff and Comaroff 2009, 46): the global indigenous people's movement; neoliberal globalization; and "previously colonized populations [who] have reversed the colonial flow from center to periphery with increased intensity, asserting their alterity, diversifying the metropole, and forcing the 'problem' of difference into the public sphere" (47).[1] With the heightened visibility of these "'others' within," health disparities have been politicized in part through the efforts of minority advocacy groups, who use health disparities claims in their demands for legal, financial, and other kinds of recognition based on ideas about cultural difference (Fraser 2001). As advocacy groups use political means to make claims based on health care inequality, health for diverse constituents is made a question of government, and new forms of biosociality (Rabinow 1996) emerge.

Building on the work of Nikolas Rose (1999) and Rose and Carlos Novas (2005), I suggest that the field of community health has contributed to the emergence of "community" as a terrain of government. In the chapters that follow, I show how community health practices contribute to both the science and art of government, as its research and programs contribute to the formation of populations such as the ethnically identified "communities" that are the focus of this work. This analysis of the concept of community at work in community health differs somewhat from that elaborated in fields such as cultural studies (e.g., Joseph 2002) or elsewhere (e.g., contributors to Creed 2006a). Miranda Joseph (2002) argues that contemporary American notions of community are supplemental to capital, fostering relationships that are meant to support consumption and supplying the social connections that capitalist society sunders. In an ethnographic analysis of San Francisco's gay community, Joseph focuses on expressions of community among predominantly white, middle-class Americans. In contrast, in community health, the concept of community signifies both minority ethnoracial identity and urban marginalization. Both Miranda Joseph and Gerald Creed, however, reveal the links among community, governance, and representation: for example, following Joseph

1. It is worth noting that oft-cited formulations of the "problem" of cultural difference, whether in the clinic, the school, or the ballot box, discursively locate the "problem" with those who are deemed "other" or different (see, for example, those introductory readers on multiculturalism and diversity with titles such as "The Challenge of Human Diversity" [Middleton 2010], "On Being Different: Diversity and Multiculturalism in the North American Mainstream" [Kottak and Kozaitis 2007], or "Understanding and Managing Diversity" [Harvey and Allard 2004]). In fact, as pointed out by many cultural competence educators who post to the Culture and Health list, the "problem" posed by the existence of the culturally different is frequently located with members of so-called mainstream or majority populations who are unable or unwilling to accommodate language or other differences in the public sphere.

(2002), Creed argues, "Community becomes more central to state governance as its political and economic power is displaced. Put more directly, communities become useful and central for the state after they have been politically eviscerated and transformed into mere units of consumption and representation. . . . To the degree that community is promoted by modern statecraft, then, it is likely to be a problematic idea of community as uniform and homogenous" (2006a, 9).

As a field of practice, community health is typically situated in urban, minority, and low-income domains and thereby embedded in the social relations that constitute experiences of race and ethnicity in the United States. At the same time, community health discourse enshrouds these contexts beneath technical concepts, approaches, practices, and models characteristic of its "parent" fields of public health and medicine. In contrast to approaches that look at community as a unit of consumption, my approach to the concept of community at work in community health is closer to that of Jenne Loyd (2010), who poses the question of "the productivity of 'community' as a material and imaginative locus for collective demands that exceed biopolitical normalization." She observes, "while practices under the banner of community health can entrench biopower, they can also serve to subvert state biopolitical practices" (40). In the following chapters, I trace the tensions invoked by these multiple capacities and the ways in which community health as a practice of governing creates new subject-positions such as "community change agent" for members of groups constituted as marginal and addressed by programs designed to mitigate this marginality.

Health Disparities, Inequality, and Neoliberalism

In the field of community health, concepts of race and ethnicity appear perhaps most frequently in assertions around *health disparities*, a term that can refer to disproportionate disease risk or outcomes among groups (e.g., Latinos are at higher risk for diabetes compared with whites; black women have higher mortality rates from breast cancer than white women, though they experience approximately the same incidence of the disease); lower rates of access to or quality of care for certain groups (e.g., Hasnain-Wynia 2010); and/or unequal life chances and life expectancy (e.g., Chapman and Berggren 2005). In its many uses and deployments, the phrase *health disparities* takes on the qualities of a floating signifier that is presumed to have both biological and social-cultural referents. Used to describe significant inequality in health status or outcomes between ethnoracial groups, the concept falls prey to contemporary confusion around—and even the rebiologization of—race and ethnicity (Epstein 2007). At the same time, the concept of health disparities allows diverse groups, including gender, sexuality, disability, and many others, to make claims regarding discrimination or inequality using the politically neutral language of health, often obscuring the racial, gendered, and economic structures of income, housing, and environment that produce disparities in the first place (Chapman and Berggren 2005).[2] The widespread use and dissemination of health disparities statements indicates the term's capaciousness, its ability to carry justice claims further, apparently, than other available discourses.[3] The language of health disparities helps propel demands made by community-based organizations onto a broader political and discursive stage, often enabling them to gain more resources and a wider audience for their work. However, efforts to eliminate the *evidence* of inequality sometimes omit concern for the causes of health disparities, such as a health system in which ability to pay determines access to and quality of care. Health disparities discourse also allows community organizations to take statements about equity that might be considered controversial, such as, "We're poor—we have no health care—we deserve better," and put them into the "objective" language of statistics and science.[4]

The concept of health disparities has emerged as a political, social, and temporal phenomenon driven by particular actors to achieve certain ends. The wide-ranging effects of this phenomenon include the generation of new forms of knowledge and the reorganization of existing forms of knowledge. Expressing political claims using the "objective" language of biomedicine and the politically neutral language of health facilitates collective action around health issues in poor and ethnically marginalized groups and simultaneously propels their claims onto a broader sociopolitical stage. By

2. Careful epidemiological studies showing the association of poor health outcomes with minority status or lower income (Krieger et al. 2005; Subramanian et al. 2005) threaten to reveal the lies that stand behind between the American ideology that "we are all equal." In fact, a thought experiment by Steven Woolf and colleagues in the *American Journal of Public Health* reported that even if the entire reduction in U.S. mortality rates between 1991 and 2000 were attributed to improvements in health care technology, which cost billions to develop, it would still be dwarfed by the number of deaths that could have been prevented if African Americans had experienced the same mortality rate as whites during the same time period (Woolf et al. 2008)—an "excess" mortality that others have argued could be solved with equality-promoting social programs costing far less than the billions spent on new health care technology.

3. Science studies theorist Bruno Latour calls such phenomena "immutable mobiles," referring to a statement's ability to be detached from its original context, transferred among multiple constituents and locations, and still retain its capacity to persuade (Latour 1988).

4. Even as the language of health disparities helps increase the political legitimacy of groups seeking to comment on their experiences of structured inequality, other political actors contest this discourse and its effectiveness in facilitating such claims. For example, the Waxman report documents the production and release of a 2003 Department of Health and Human Services analysis of health disparities in the United States that was effectively censored by the second Bush administration in order to minimize the assessment of U.S. health disparities. The Democrats' Special Investigations Division uncovered the manipulation of the report and forced the release of the original unmodified draft (Wright 2007).

using health issues to stake claims regarding marginalization and to pose demands for resources, poor and ethnically marginalized groups are thus able to depoliticize a thorny social problem as they appeal to and in some cases appropriate biomedical knowledge and expertise (Epstein 2007). The aim of this project, then, is to *repoliticize* this depoliticized effort.

In his book *Inclusion: The Politics of Difference in Medical Research* (2007), Steven Epstein traces the emergence and unintended consequences of one set of policy remedies for health disparities, those requiring the inclusion of women and people of color in federally funded clinical research. Technologies of culturally appropriate health care, discussed in Chapter 4, are another set of changes to health care that, with the advent of federal regulations, is slowly moving toward becoming established health care policy.[5] Hospital administrators, primary care clinics, and even emergency departments are seeking to modify their business practices to emulate the goal of culturally and linguistically appropriate services. This process is simultaneously being administered from the upper reaches of health care policy at the same time as it is actively lobbied for by minority nongovernmental organizations such as the health center where my fieldwork was based (Shaw 2001). How do these fields of contestation around managing difference in health care intersect with state and other efforts to regulate the health and behavior of low-income and marginalized populations? Chapter 4 explores the ways in which cultural expertise is being commodified and disseminated by cultural competence trainers, minority health advocates, and others. Organizing efforts around culturally appropriate health care bring together a wide range of actors and advocates seeking to reform health care, including refugee aid organizations, people interested in patient-centered health care, and antiracism activists, among others. At the same time, culturally appropriate health care efforts take place in health care environments increasingly concerned with cost-effectiveness and "doing more with less."

Neoliberal reforms devolve responsibility to nongovernmental actors for previously governmental functions to form what Suzan Ilcan and Tanya Basok call "community government" (2004). Neoliberal developments have fundamentally reshaped public health and primary health care in the United States as market rationalities of efficiency, accountability, and productivity are extended into social domains previously associated with social norms such as equality or justice (Ong 2006; Briggs and Hallin

---

5. For example, see the national standards for culturally and linguistically appropriate services, known as the CLAS standards, published in the *Federal Register* on December 22, 2000 (vol. 65, no. 247, pp. 80865–80879). The CLAS standards appear in their entirety on the U.S. Office of Minority Health (OMH) Web site, http://minorityhealth.hhs.gov/templates/browse.aspx?lvl=2&lvlid=15. The CLAS standards have recently been incorporated into the guidelines used by Joint Commission surveyors in their annual reviews of health care organizations; see Chapter 4.

2007). Neoliberal reforms institute new regimes of government, for both programs and individuals, by changing the rules, outcomes, and processes of governance through the provision of services. New forms of account-ability demand more and more businesslike approaches to such humanitar-ian projects as soup kitchens and literacy programs. Neoliberal solutions to the putative problems of "big government" offer not only to make government smaller but also to manage it like a business, governed by prin-ciples of competition, the logic of the market, and demands of customers (Clarke 2007). Big government, exemplified by a U.S. welfare system seen as rambling, inefficient, and inaccurate, was a prominent rationale cited in both the 1995–1996 welfare debate and in more recent opposition to the Obama administration's health care reform effort of 2010. The 1996 welfare reform law, and similar efforts in Great Britain and Australia (e.g., Clarke 2008; Dean 1997), sought to better administer the welfare system through privatization.

Locating responsibility for social problems such as poverty within the bodies of the poor, neoliberal social policy seeks to reform the conduct of the poor by connecting it up with the interests of society (Rose 1999). Feminist theorists and researchers point out that the bodies of the poor are always gendered and that women's bodies are often subject to greater control and surveillance than men's (Abramovitz 1988; Campbell 2000). Though the 1996 welfare reform act was in large part directed at the government of poor women, its programs attack the notion of gender as a primary analytic construct, focusing instead on gender-neutral notions of "productivity" and "parenting." Welfare reform—making women into workers—is a matter of giving lessons in citizenship to poor women, par-ticularly to women of color.[6] Broader transformations associated with neo-liberalism foreground ethnicity through the language of community, while gender is pushed to the back as women are made into good mothers in the battle against dependency by becoming good workers.[7] In my fieldwork, despite being everywhere present and enacted, gender was oddly absent from the rhetorical framework used to mobilize citizens through the notion of community. Similarly, in much public health literature, "community" is used in place of or to stand for ethnicity, ethnic identity, or ethnic groups—that is, to refer to people of color and seldom to people of Euro-American

---

6. Describing a case where the (lack of) citizenship is at issue for undocumented parents and their children, Sarah Horton and Judith Barker (2009) discuss the roles of public health workers as intermediaries and civilizing agents for immigrant populations whose children have serious oral health problems.

7. Many have pointed out the double standard here between poor women, who provide a good example for their children by working outside the home to become self-sufficient, and middle- and upper-class women who stay at home to raise their children to provide them the best opportunities offered by a (middle-class) mother's time and attention.

or "white" ethnicity.[8] Part I of this book describes ways in which notions of community are linked to ethnicity through technical and administrative practices, as well as through community organizing efforts that function as practices of identity.

Routes of Contest: Governmental and Other Representations of Ethnicity

Marisol de la Cadena (2000) emphasizes that collectively defined meanings of race and ethnicity are always the outcome of political struggle. In the field of community health, struggles take place using resources made available through discursive conflicts; as Pierre Bourdieu suggests, groups are able to use only the resources they have secured through previous struggles (1991). My own interest in discussing ethnicity is not so much to account for where these notions of ethnic differences come from but rather what they mean in practices of community health and research, and how notions of ethnicity are mobilized as resources in particular social, institutional, and economic circumstances.[9] As shown in greater detail in Chapter 2, meanings of ethnicity and community interlock with urban practices of segregation to buttress claims from local agencies that they "represented" specific "communities." I describe the ways in which agencies and groups in Thornton used practices of ethnic identification as a means by which to make claims for social justice and entitlement.

In their book *Ethnicity, Inc.*, John and Jean Comaroff define ethnicity as

> neither a monolithic "thing" nor, in and of itself, an analytic con struct: [rather,] "it" is best understood as a loose, labile repertoire of signs by means of which relations are constructed and communicated; through which a collective consciousness of cultural likeness is rendered sensible; with reference to which shared sentiment is made substantial. Its visible content is *always* a product of specific historical conditions which, in variable measure, impinge themselves on human perception and, in so doing, frame the motivation, meaning and materiality of social practice. (2009, 38)

Throughout this book, I use the term *ethnicity* to refer to an individual's ethnic identity, as well as to the structures of identification that

---

8. In her ethnography of a U.S. high school, Mica Pollock describes a similar process in which arguments about education disparities among students, teachers, and policy makers did and did not draw on what she terms "race labels" (Pollock 2005, 8).
9. But on the social production of racial categories, see also Clarke and Thomas 2006, Briggs 2004, Crenshaw et al. 1995, Frankenberg 1993, Jewett 2006, Omi and Winant 1989, and Santiago-Irizarry 2001, among others.

characterize collective references to groups of people according to cultural or national background. In this way, ethnicity became an important problematic in this project.[10] Similarly, in conversations that took place during my fieldwork in Thornton, the term *community* was used to refer to both specific and general collectivities of people, geographic areas, laypeople as opposed to professionals, and people of color both in general and in particular. After giving a brief overview of governmental technologies of racial and ethnic classification, I turn to the impact of health disparities discourse on individual and community mobilization.

In addition to providing locally significant structures of meaning for people in Thornton and elsewhere, ethnic categories are an important tool in governing.[11] The collection of data about populations is an important function of government since "data gathered by race and ethnicity are used in public health to set goals, establish programs and policies, and measure progress" (Sondik et al. 2000, 1711). Medical anthropologists, public health researchers, and many others mobilize statistics to document health disparities but are often foiled in their efforts by the multiple possible referents of the terms *race* and *ethnicity*. Public health researchers and others concerned with health disparities spend a lot of time discussing the best way to collect such information. As one hospital administrator wrote to the Culture and Health list, "valid and reliable patient demographic data on race, ethnicity and language [is a primary need], recognizing that this should be a foundation of all efforts toward measuring and reducing health disparities and building cultural competence."[12] However, the on-the-ground complexity of this apparently straightforward administrative

---

10. Interestingly, while the Comaroffs observe that "ethnicity—like 'identity,' with which it is often twinned—has become a taken-for-granted usage in the argot of everyday life across the planet" (2009, 38), in my own fieldwork, whenever I asked low-income African Americans and Puerto Ricans in Thornton to name their ethnicity for quantitative surveys, I usually had to give them a prompt: "You know, like black, white, Latino." This experience raises the question: How taken for granted is it, in what ways, and for whom?

11. See also the May 2010 special issue of *Anthropology News* on cross-cultural studies of census technologies.

12. Postings to this e-mail list are discussed in greater detail in Chapter 4. A fascinating area for further research would be a cross-cultural comparison of uses of the concept of "health disparities" or comparable ideas. For example, Francois Héran, director of France's Institut National d'Etudes Demographiques argued that France has no history of discrimination, and he further asserted that universal health insurance should erase any ethnic differences in health status or outcomes. French health disparities researchers feel that ethnic categories have *less* explanatory power (in part because of concern about levels of aggregation: Which groups are combined to create the category "African"? What differences are obscured by that category?) than what they call *trajectories de precarité*, or "trajectories/careers of vulnerability." (From field notes taken at a conference organized by the Working Group on Health Disparities at the Harvard School of Public Health, "Making Disparities Count: From Government Statistics Systems to Action," Cambridge, Massachusetts, May 5, 2005. For an official summary of the conference, see http://134.174.190.199/disparities/book/HealthDisparities.pdf.)

challenge highlights the instability of racial-ethnic categories (Takeuchi and Gage 2003; Dressler, Oths, and Gravlee 2005) that are used in medical and public health research: How are language groups identified and aggregated? How is ethnicity categorized? Will we follow the U.S. census division between racial and ethnic categories? How will immigrant groups be accounted for? What is meant by *race*? By *ethnicity*?

"Racial" and "ethnic" populations are constituted according to ever-shifting categories elaborated in governmental technologies such as the census, itself a product of ongoing negotiation and struggle (Wallman, Evinger, and Schechter 2000). Sociologist of science Steven Epstein provides a careful review and discussion of the changes to the U.S. census between 1990 and 2000 after extensive debate about the validity of categories of race and ethnicity used therein (Epstein 2007).[13] People participate in discourses of ethnicity through practices of identification in which the terms and conditions of belonging are elaborated in technologies such as the census. The census thus constitutes new groups and populations,[14] even as its categories are variously mobilized and contested by members advancing their social agendas. Preexisting relations of ethnic identity and belonging, and their conscription by states as statistics later used to document health disparities, have been critical to community health programs as states seek to mobilize the bonds and, at times, the divisions of ethnicity in delivering services.

The response from public health scholars and practitioners to these changes in the 2000 census reveals the political importance of the categorization of ethnicity for governing health. Public health researchers and advocates have clashed over the use and deployment of ethnoracial categories as a means to track inequality. While the Office of Management and Budget (OMB), in its federal mandate on the collection of racial/ethnic data known as OMB Statistical Directive 15, acknowledges that "the categories in this classification are social-political constructs and should not be interpreted as being scientific or anthropological in nature" (Wallman, Evinger, and Schechter 2000, 1706), many argue that any classification of people by race nonetheless perpetuates its reification. The Institute of Medicine has suggested that race be eliminated from census categories and replaced by ethnicity, while others in public health believe that the elimination of race as a category of analysis would rule out the ability to track empirically "the existence and consequences of racism, including its impact on health" (Oppenheimer 2001, 1053). For example, an epidemiologist writing in the American Journal of Public Health argues that "by taking

---

13. See also Bliss 2009 and 2010, Fausto-Sterling 2004, Sondik et al. 2000, and contributors to the *Anthropology News* special issue on technologies of the census (May 2010).
14. See Igo 2007 for a related discussion of the role of public opinion polls in constructing the self-identity of residents of "Middletown, USA."

away the ability to link health status and race, we remove one of the most powerful tools used by disenfranchised people to fight for social justice, not only in medical care and public health, but also in our development as a nation" (Thomas 2001, 1047).[15] This contest hints at both the stakes involved in the social production of racial classification and the centrality of practices of racial classification for governing projects.[16] While these authors focus on race in their discussions of health disparities, throughout this book I follow cultural anthropological convention and discuss ascribed population differences as ethnicity (e.g., Montoya 2007) in my analyses of these and other struggles in community health.

Howard Winant (1994) reminds us that ethnic identities function as a structuring force of social relations in the United States. In *The Black Atlantic*, Paul Gilroy proposes the notion of "routes" over the more conventional understanding of "roots" as a productive way to develop a liberatory understanding of ethnicity (1993). Gilroy describes "the history of the black Atlantic . . . , continually crisscrossed by the movements of black people—not only as commodities but engaged in various struggles towards emancipation, autonomy, and citizenship" to provide a setting for his examination of "the problems of nationality, location, identity, and historical memory" (Gilroy 1993, 16). In a critique of U.S. black nationalists, he observes that "modern black political culture has always been more interested in the relationship of identity to roots and rootedness than in seeing identity as a process of movement and mediation that is more appropriately approached via the homonym routes" (Gilroy 1993, 19). I want to retain the performative and active sense of "routes" as I look at the discourses of ethnicity and community that emerged in and around community health practices in Thornton and elsewhere. As he works out an anti-essentialist understanding of culture and identity, Gilroy asserts that blackness is more "a matter of politics rather than a common cultural condition" (1993, 27). If politics is understood as "all deliberate efforts to control shared systems of meaning" (Sederberg, qtd. in B. Williams 1991, 269), then we can look at struggles over health, identity, and legitimacy as arenas in which the meaning of ethnicity was elaborated, controlled, and mobilized. Naming health challenges for specific ethnoracial groups "health disparities," and identifying solutions based on these categories of belonging, is a way of instrumentalizing the social relations that make up ethnic categories and identification. Peter Sederberg's definition extends colloquial understandings of politics to encompass dimensions of meaning-making that are active in and critical to projects of governing through community health. Though

---

15. See Jewett 2006 for a cogent, ethnographically based discussion of the bureaucratic production and uses of racial categories in middle school.
16. For further related discussions, see Dressler et al. 2005, Fullwiley 2007, Gravlee and Sweet 2008, Kahn 2006, Lee 2005, and Montoya 2007.

community health has always been a site of tension between professional and anti-establishment forces, shared systems of meanings are created and circulated within its disciplinary boundaries, made up of elements of public health, social medicine, and primary health care.

Biocitizenship and Biosociality: Making Up Community Health

These local and dispersed struggles over community health offer several paths by which we may explore the diverse meanings of governance, citizenship, and identity formation. Actors as varied as community-based organizations and hospital administrators draw on discourses of rights and responsibilities in their efforts to determine whether and how to provide health care within terms set by state policies addressing access and citizenship. Concepts of health and illness both mediate and facilitate claims on the state for benefits, entitlements, and recognition (Petryna 2002; Rose 2006; Fairchild, Bayer, and Colgrove 2007, ch. 5), serving as universal values (Laclau 1995) that help produce new forms of community and sociality.

Anthropologists have used the concept of *biocitizenship* to variously describe the obligations around health promotion assigned to active citizens, the transfer of responsibility for health from the state to citizen-subjects (Briggs and Hallin 2007), and the use of bodily affliction to facilitate claims on the state (Petryna 2002). Certain populations inhabiting the margins of U.S. society are among those whose attenuated claims on the state are mediated by demonstrable embodied harm (see Biehl 2005). Outlining the ways in which liberal conceptions of citizenship are fragmenting among migrant and stateless populations in transnational economies, Aihwa Ong (2006) offers a critique of Giorgio Agamben's concept of "bare life" that seeks to overcome the opposition between the excluded and the included in political discourse. Ong writes, "A strict adherence to Agamben's universal division of humanity into those with rights and those without would miss the rich complexity and the possibilities of multiple ethical systems at play" (23). Instead, Ong seeks to discover the ways in which humanity and citizenship are contested and constructed depending on local conditions, economies, and identity formations. Ong continues, "Agamben's fundamental reference of bare life in a state of permanent exception thus ignores the possibility of complex negotiations of claims for those without territorialized citizenship" (23). The case studies discussed here represent a series of complex negotiations of claims using the vehicle of community health knowledge and practices. In diverse domains, citizenship is produced and contested as marginalized groups bump up against various state apparatuses bent on simultaneously ignoring and managing their existence.

When community organizations in the United States offer resources and services to injection drug users "at risk" for HIV, for example, what Ong refers to as "the nonstate administration of excluded humanity" (2006, 24) flourishes. Like the radiation victims described by Adriana Petryna (2002) or the people living with AIDS portrayed by Joao Biehl (2004), community health and advocacy groups for the minority poor in the United States seek rights and entitlements based on health status, creating forms of biocitizenship that mitigate against the structural exclusion of minority and low-income populations most at risk for HIV infection and other negative health outcomes. Illicit drug users are among those most likely to be excluded from the rights and benefits of citizenship; once convicted of a felony, they lose federal housing and education benefits for which they might otherwise be income-eligible, as well as, often, lifetime suffrage (Mauer and Chesney-Lind 2002).[17] Part II of this book explores the complex modes of governing that help construct and manage this excluded population, including publicly funded public health research and HIV prevention programs.

And yet marginalized groups are also engaged in developing programs for themselves, such as the outreach worker program described in Chapters 2 and 3, or the syringe exchange program described in Chapter 6, as part of the process of instantiating themselves as political subjects as well as the objects of intervention. Biosociality posits that new forms of social relations and identities emerge as people integrate health information into their understandings of themselves and their relations with others (e.g., Ong and Collier 2005; Rabinow 1996; Rose and Novas 2005). This project extends the concept of biosociality from the level of individual biology (e.g., Taussig, Heath, and Rapp 2003) into new domains such as access to health care populated by low-income and marginalized members of U.S. society. As groups organize around issues of importance to them— gender discrimination, AIDS, or poverty, for example—their collective action provides the spark that leads to the emergence of new identities such as feminist or AIDS activist (D'Emilio 2003; Morgen 2002; Mercer 1994; Klawiter 2008). At the same time, collective action around community health also develops as the result of transformations in individual

---

17. One service provider I interviewed observed, "In this state now, if you have a CORI [Criminal Offender Record Information, a public record of every criminal court appearance by an individual], and I don't know an addict who doesn't, you're not eligible for higher ed, you're not eligible for low-income housing, you're not eligible for a lot of jobs. . . . There are a lot of folks who don't even qualify for public assistance because of their CORI. And so if you have no money, no job, no hope for improvement so that you can move to another state, . . . then you have no other recourse but to do what you know how to do. And survival has a lot of faces."

and collective identity (Klawiter 2008; see also Escobar, Rocheleau, and Kothari 2002).[18]

Popular and policy discourses typically construct the ethnically and economically marginalized as a problem for governing, as criminalized or excluded from political processes. My ethnographic research reveals, in contrast, that members of these groups use a variety of means to organize around health issues, both contesting and inhabiting identity categories as they engage in practices of self-governing. Advocacy groups may seize on infant mortality rates, for example, as an opportunity for the construction of new forms of identity and concomitant claims for recognition (Shaw 2005). In Thornton and elsewhere, individual and collective identities are shaped by the intersection of white privilege with advanced marginalization, defining white suburban voters as citizens while residents of the inner city core are viewed as recipients of services. These hierarchies of privilege also determine structural and policy responses to public health crises such as the HIV epidemic (Shaw 2006; Biehl 2005). In community health settings, biosociality extends beyond genes or disease in individual bodies to describe the ways in which economically and ethnically diverse actors understand and act on health issues to comment on their community's marginalization and to make claims on the state. New forms of politicized identities ensue.

If public health is about the government of populations, both in the sense of maintaining a healthy population (Foucault 1991) and in the sense of ensuring the equitable distribution of health resources, then it is a technique of biopower. Public health programs are also a way for citizens and communities, in advocating for or contesting such resources, to express their visions of what constitutes a just society or the social good. For example, state-sponsored HIV prevention programs such as syringe exchange for injection drug users, which some view as condoning drug use, thus become sites where citizens' understandings of who may count as a member of "the public" rubs up uncomfortably against others' views of what constitutes "justice" (Shaw 2006). Further, technologies of government such as the Community Health Advocate (CHA) program were

---

18. Robert Lorway and colleagues analyze an empowerment program for male sex workers in Mysore, India, and trace the emergence of new forms of subjectivity among its participants. They write, "An understanding of male sex work, in the case of our study, requires examination of the subjectivities and social relations that form within the discursive terrain where 'sex work,' 'sexual risk,' and 'self-empowerment' assemble under the banner of epidemic prevention. In other words, this article attempts to reveal how the category 'male sex worker' allows certain individuals to remember their sense of sexual-gender difference into unfolding narratives of becoming for the purpose of political mobilization" (Lorway, Reza-Paul, and Pasha 2009, 143).

developed to create communities as political subjects and to allow groups of people to constitute themselves as a public (Klawiter 2008).

Thinking through Difference

Governmentality, while revealing certain processes, obscures others. Governmentality helps us rearticulate questions of public health as questions of government and can allow us to better understand the difficulties faced by AIDS prevention programs, for example, that provide heroin addicts with sterile syringes (as discussed in Chapter 6). Governmentality allows us to perceive the range of resources that are available to actors struggling with the regulation of conduct. Yet with these optics come limitations; for example, governmentality may eclipse the nuanced social contexts in which practices of government take place, concealing the means through which certain populations are defined as valuable or worth intervention, while others may be discarded (Fassin 2007). The all-encompassing logic of governmentality theory, in the hands of some, can obscure the complex and varied conditions under which people engage or refuse to participate in practices of self-government, "presenting the reproduction of power relations as a [uniform] matter of *social control*" (Barnett 2005, 9). Governmentality theory often fails to ask questions about individual experience or motivation, frequently paying little attention to the formation of subjectivities (Barnett 2005).[19] Similarly, an attention to culture as the lived, contested social environment in which thought and action take place is rather notoriously absent (Bennett 2003), though this is lately being remedied (see, e.g., Biehl 2005).

I draw on both political-economic approaches and post-structuralist theories of governmentality in this analysis. Governmentality theories allow me to attend to community health as *both* a means by which marginalized groups organize for the more equitable distribution of resources *and* part of the governing assemblage that manages, constrains, and diffuses the concerns of such groups and the effectiveness of their mobilization. At the same time, I am politically and ethically compelled by the promise of what David Harvey calls "embedded liberalism," seen, for example (at least formerly), in European social welfare states (Navarro 2004): the belief that "the state should focus on full employment, economic growth, and the welfare of its citizens, and that state power should be freely deployed, alongside of or . . . even substituting for market processes to achieve these ends" (Harvey 2005, 11). While to me, governmentality is better able to explain the liberatory practices of those with whom I worked (deploying categories of knowledge and identity to obtain greater

---

19. But for exceptions, see Reardon 2005, Taussig et al. 2003, and Sharma 2008, among others.

resources and better political representation), political economy provides the more convincing accounting of the unequal distribution of health and illness in the United States that follows from the extraction of profit in capitalist democracy.

According to political economists such as David Harvey, the role of the state in neoliberalism is to facilitate the transfer of wealth and income from lower classes to upper classes (2005). In his *Brief History of Neoliberalism* (2005), Harvey suggests:

> Neoliberalism is in the first instance a theory of political economic practices that proposes that human well-being can best be advanced by liberating individual entrepreneurial freedoms and skills within an institutional framework characterized by strong private property rights, free markets, and free trade. The role of the state is to create and preserve an institutional framework appropriate to such practices. . . . Furthermore, if markets do not exist (in areas such as land, water, education, health care, social security, or environmental pollution) then they must be created, by state action if necessary. But beyond these tasks the state should not venture. (2)

Political economists look at welfare as a means of maintaining the "reserve labor force" at minimal levels of subsistence, while governmentality theorists emphasize instead the role of self-governance enacted in Welfare-to-Work (WtW) and similar programs (see Chapter 4). According to David Harvey, the "social good," for neoliberals, is achieved through the marketization of "all human action" (2005, 3), while in the hands of governmentality theorists "the good" is achieved by rationalizing power and linking individual interests with those of the state (or the market) (Rose 1999; Dean 1999). What Harvey calls the "neoliberal state" (2005, 7) is one that supports these aims through individual property rights, "freely negotiated contractual obligations between juridical individuals in the marketplace," markets unencumbered by regulation or trade restrictions, and the "rule of law" (64; see also Goode and Maskovsky 2001). In contrast, governmentality theorists focus on the circulation of power and the constitution of subjects. They are less concerned with the transfer of wealth from working to ruling classes than with "the well-being of populations" (Li 2007, 12, citing Foucault) and describing the relocation of techniques of power from the state to citizen-subjects (Rose 1999). In representative democracy, government's legitimacy is attained from those who are governed. In contrast to analyses of neoliberalism based on Marxist political economy, Foucaultian approaches to government look at the way that power constitutes subjects. Systems of classification and knowledge production are as important, in this approach, as types of government or economy (Dean 1999; Ferguson and Gupta 2002).

Despite their many differences, theorists of political economy and governmentality share some critiques of modern governing (Barnett 2005; Li 2007). Both political economists and governmentality theorists point to the emergence of government by experts and the new configurations of expertise that result. While governmentality theorists focus on the transfer of power and authority from the state to citizen-subjects, David Harvey argues that

> neoliberal theorists are . . . profoundly suspicious of democracy. Governance by majority rule is seen as a potential threat to individual rights and constitutional liberties. Democracy is viewed as a luxury, only possible under conditions of relative affluence coupled with a strong middle-class presence to guarantee political stability. Neoliberals therefore tend to favour governance by experts and elites. . . . This creates the paradox of intense state interventions [in setting up markets] and government by elites in a world where the state is supposed to not be interventionist. (2005, 66, 69)

According to governmentality theorists, in contrast, assemblages that unite states with nonstate actors such as nongovernmental organizations (NGOs) and multilateral organizations such as the World Bank mobilize and contest expertise in the process of constructing and governing populations. Anthony Giddens argues that amid the uncertainty of late modernity, governing at a distance takes place through experts who win "collective trust" and thereby the consent of the governed (Michael 1996, 574; Giddens 1994). Experts produce and circulate "legitimatory discourses" that enable dispersed modes of surveillance and social control (Michael 1996, 576).

Both political economists and governmentality theorists analyze the entrepreneurialization of government that permeates public-private partnerships such as WtW (Larner 2005). Both schools of thought hold that under neoliberalism, the state increasingly assigns responsibility for well-being to individuals (Goode and Maskovsky 2001; Bunton 2005). Finally, both political economy and governmentality theorists point to the ever-increasing role of NGOs as a key tool of governance; for example, David Harvey points out the shift to "governance (a broader configuration of state and key elements in civil society)" through the widespread emergence of public-private partnerships (2005, 77). Many emphasize the ways in which advocacy groups have proliferated under neoliberalism (Harvey 2005, 77), at times accelerating state withdrawal from social service provision as they step in to fill the gap (Harvey 2005, 177).

As emphasized by Barbara Cruikshank (1999), Aradhana Sharma (2008), and others, programs aimed at "empowerment," such as the CHA program or harm reduction programs for drug users, are always already relations of power. In a range of arenas from community health in the United States to international health and development, empowerment programs seek to shape political subjects into citizens (e.g., Lorway, Reza-Paul, and Pasha 2009). Do programs aimed at empowerment have a greater chance of "success," however defined, than more authoritarian or didactic programs that place less credence in the knowledge and abilities of the people being "empowered"? I believe they do, in part because of my political beliefs in the importance of self-determination and in part because evidence suggests that people do better when treated as peers or equals rather than as pupils.[20] However, I am not sure this is the most important question to ask. Instead, we may do better to focus on the ways in which programs and activities such as syringe exchange and cultural competency trainings constitute new kinds of subjects that both take part in and resist new modes of governing. Governmentality shows us how the pragmatics of government are ethical and teleological: the government of populations takes place on the grounds of what is good or right.[21] From this starting point, we can look at public health programs as techniques of citizenship—a way of organizing power in which states seek to produce subjects who are active rather than apathetic participants in the project of governing (Cruikshank 1999)—that shape who and what public health workers (including primary care physicians, CHAs, and syringe exchange workers) should be, by producing new subject-positions embedded in complex assemblages of knowledge and practice.

Empowerment-based programs often depend on, if not require, the direct participation of the marginalized populations who are their target. Authentic participation easily translates into policy solutions based on "self sufficiency" because the same politics of voice that demands that the poor be empowered to "speak for themselves" also emphasizes their "own" resources and capacities in discourses of self-sufficiency.[22] The question posed by governmentality, then, concerns the ways in which programs such as CHAs or syringe exchange for injection drug users also serve as the means of governing the poor. Governmentality raises questions of theory and practice because it is about the application of knowledge: "Thus to analyse mentalities of government is to analyse thought made practical and

---

20. See, for example, Beam and Tessaro 1994, Breines 1989, Braithwaite et al. 1989, and Broadhead and Fox 1990.

21. "The policies and practices of government . . . presume to know, . . . using specific forms of knowledge, what constitutes good, virtuous, appropriate, responsible conduct of individual and collectivities. [Government is] an attempt to shape who and what we should be" (Dean 1999, 12).

22. As Chris Miller and Yusuf Ahmad observe, "The ethic of self-help, and the attack on an apparent dependency culture [of welfare], has ensured the transference of the burden of care from state agencies to the non-profit, community and informal, as well as private, sectors" (1997, 271).

technical" (Dean 1999, 18). These questions highlight the ethics of how programmers and analysts think about cultural difference in health care.

Public health programs, including the CHA program and cultural competency training efforts for health care providers, rely on the authenticity of their community members to mobilize funding resources and justify interventions. In sometimes unforeseen ways, discourses of identity, belonging, and authenticity can form boundaries to restrict the paths that agencies can take and shape the programs that govern the poor. Chapter 2 describes the ways in which CHA leaders fostered an "analysis of oppression" that integrates, yet seeks to act within, the tension between an understanding of actors as fully endowed agents capable of agitating for and bringing about change, and an insistence on the social, political, and economic forces that constrain the choices actors make. This tension, revealed in the kinds of programmatic solutions discussed here, locates the CHA program squarely within unresolved questions of agency, politics, and government.

I

Technologies of Citizenship and Difference

L ong concerned with urban, low-income, and marginalized populations, community health workers and scholars use a range of strategies to highlight ethnic and racial health disparities and engage diverse groups in programs to improve health. These strategies and programs respond to the social construction of difference as expressed in statements about unequal health outcomes among ethnic groups. Community health researchers collaborate with those seeking to reform medical education and health care to eliminate disparities in care; both groups draw on constructions of difference and meanings of recognition as they construct their target populations. In both cases that make up this section, programs developed to implement social justice ideals wind up producing in practice essentialized or otherwise problematic understandings of difference. In each case presented here, diverse actors, including community health activists, health care administrators, and antiracist educators, develop responses to problems of difference and distance between service providers and patients—responses that carry a range of unintended effects (Li 2007).

Two studies make up this section concerned with technologies of citizenship and difference. The first case study analyzes how social differences between white health care providers and patients who are people of color were addressed by recruiting African American and Latina welfare recipients as outreach workers, called Community Health Advocates (CHAs), for a group of three Thornton agencies. These CHAs were meant to enroll "hard to serve" minority and inner-city residents as patients at Thornton Community Health Center (TCHC) and its two partner agencies. Concepts of difference permeated the program: ethnic identity was woven into the notion of "community" through the practices and rhetoric of the empowerment model. At the same time, the language of empowerment that drove the program translated with disconcerting ease into concepts of self-sufficiency characteristic of neoliberal modes of governing. Chapters 2 and 3 discuss the changes as well as continuities in the CHA program when, midway through my fieldwork, it received federal welfare reform funding. In the aftermath, we see the unexpected ways in which community empowerment is consonant with the ideologies and practices of neoliberal government, as well as the heavy costs to TCHC staff and the CHA participants associated with this new funding source.

The second case study presented in this section builds on what I learned when I talked to patients and health care providers at TCHC about what makes health care culturally appropriate (Shaw 2001, 2005, 2010). Chapter 4 pulls our ethnographic focus up from local culturally appropriate health care programs to examine efforts by hospitals and health care providers across the United States to enact a set of regulations and guidelines for culturally and linguistically appropriate services (the CLAS standards) issued by the U.S. Office of Minority Health in 2001. Chapter 4 analyzes postings to an e-mail discussion list for health care administrators and my field notes and transcripts from face-to-face conferences to explore ethical-political solutions to the "problem" of cultural difference in health care. In response to calls for tailoring health care to the needs of diverse ethnic groups, a new knowledge formation, "culturally appropriate health care," has emerged as an important site for the construction and negotiation of cultural difference. Minority and other nongovernmental organizations have mobilized around the concept of culture in health, contributing to a range of curricula, tools, trainings, and guides for health care providers. These tools function as new social technologies that increase the legitimacy of marginalized forms of expertise and modify doctor-patient interactions in order to produce more equal health outcomes.

Both the lay health outreach worker program analyzed in Chapters 2 and 3 and the online trainings for physicians seen in Chapter 4 offer different means of negotiating difference in the clinic. As "providers of last resort" for the poor, community health centers have long cared for predominantly minority patient populations, especially in urban areas (Loyd 2010). Initiated as a means of bridging a racialized gap (that is often discussed in terms of "culture") between TCHC staff and residents of its surrounding neighborhoods, the CHA program found itself managing and serving the poor and minority women who signed up to be CHAs when it received Welfare-to-Work (WtW) funding. Chapters 2 and 3 explore the apparent puzzle of two very different approaches to the government of the poor coexisting within one community health program that was supposedly aimed at their empowerment. Eventually I realized that these two approaches were not so different; they shared characteristics of language and structure. Each approach relied on certain shared political assumptions that allowed them to both momentarily "drive" the same program. The WtW and empowerment approaches were both built around an autonomous actor, for example, who either worked on herself to become a productive citizen or worked on her community to constitute it as a political subject. Both approaches held a vision of the social good that animated, mobilized, or justified their methods. Both saw "the community" as in need in relation to the larger society. These similarities reveal the function of community empowerment as a technique of government, one of whose aims is the mobilization of difference in order to overcome gaps imposed by the structural marginalization of racialized and impoverished urban citizen-subjects.

Various conditions of possibility allow the language of community and empowerment to be adopted and adapted by conservative social reformers. In Part II I suggest that the "empowerment" approach to the CHA program discussed in Chapter 2 operated via the same types of productive, disciplinary practices as the more explicitly job training–oriented program discussed in Chapter 3. This part presents those conditions of possibility in an analysis of changes in social and health policy associated with neoliberalism in the United States in the late 1980s and 1990s. To help us understand these changes, I use the framework of governmentality developed by Michel Foucault and elaborated on by several social theorists, notably Nikolas Rose (1999), Peter Miller (1995), Barbara Cruikshank (1999), and others. I demonstrate through a study of public health and social work practices how contradictions between two quite different approaches (WtW and empowerment) to the CHA program were both resolved and sustained through the shared capacities of the language of empowerment, community, and health. Similar contradictions can be found in culturally appropriate health care (CAHC) programs, as representatives of empowered communities contribute to essentialized representations of culture, ethnicity, or difference that contravene their understandings of individualized, patient-centered health care.

To be effective, both CAHC and public health outreach programs depend on and construct particular kinds of populations. Michel Foucault locates the possibility of democratic government in the identification and comprehension of populations (1991). Modern government requires the gathering of knowledge of the assembled subjects who make up populations. The mobilization and application of that knowledge is an integral part of the exercise of power. Public health, a set of techniques for more equitably distributing health resources throughout a population, is also a means of governing populations (Gastaldo 1997). Public health both designates and controls populations; at the same time, groups use both public health statistics and public health organizations like Thornton Community

Health Center to represent their concerns to the state. For example, communities seeking to constitute themselves as political actors make political claims using health status as evidence for their argument (such as that poor communities have higher mortality rates, HIV rates, or smoking rates). Public health provides a readily available language for this sort of tactic (see, e.g., Epstein 2007; Metcalfe 1993).

At the level of individual subjects, theories of governmentality allow me to analyze the ways in which the new subject-position "Community Health Advocates"—low-income women of color who are trained to do door-to-door outreach—emerges from two quite different techniques of government: community development training and WtW training. The lines of this argument follow in some ways that of Akhil Gupta and Aradhana Sharma, except that Gupta and Sharma outline the similar outcomes of two separate programs "embodying very different ideologies and goals" (Gupta and Sharma 2006, 277), as a means of showing the coherence in practice despite transformations in governing ideologies. In contrast, I track the transformations and consistency of one program under two different funding mechanisms over a briefer period of time.

Building from a description of the specific meanings of "citizen" and "subject" in political science, Barbara Cruikshank proposes a new form of political subject, the "citizen-subject" (1999). This "hybrid" actor is defined through the relationship implied by the hyphen between forces of domination and agency—the citizen-subject comes to the fore to aid in our understanding of, especially, participatory democracy.[1] This figure is particularly helpful as we look at the overlap between two different discourses that share the same political end: the formation of *active* and *self-governing* subjects. A technology of citizenship is one means of constructing self-governing subjects. Technologies of citizenship do not function only by means of repression, in other words. Cruikshank emphasizes that this concept of the citizen-subject was derived from the continuing push for *participation* in programs such as the CHA program. She notes that community development programs can be seen as "a method for constituting citizens out of subjects and maximizing their political participation" (1999, 67).

These discussions rely on current efforts in anthropology, sociology, and elsewhere in the social sciences to analyze practices of government as regimes of power. The use of welfare recipients as lay health outreach workers to deliver the "message" of empowerment to the inner-city poor is embedded in broader practices of community health, as is the circulation of

---

1. "In short, I am suggesting that if power is not external to the state of being citizen or subject, if to be self-governing is to be both citizen and subject, both subject to and the subject of government, then a welfare recipient, for example, is not the antithesis of an active citizen" (Cruikshank 1999, 23).

discourses of equality through online media and face-to-face interventions for health care providers. These technologies of government subsume an understanding of gender, health, and welfare beneath discourses of community and ethnic identity.[2] Governmentality focuses our attention on the extension of state powers into new realms of social and economic life through complex assemblages of actors and organizations, including CHAs, the agencies who sponsor them, hospital administrators, federal regulators, and the physicians who enroll in cultural competency trainings to learn how to provide culturally appropriate health care.

---

2. A technology of government "is an assemblage of forms of practical knowledge, with modes of perception, practices of calculation, vocabularies, types of authority, forms of judgment, architectural forms, human capacity . . . and so forth, traversed and transected by aspirations to achieve certain outcomes in terms of the conduct of the governed" (Rose 1999, 52).

2

Community Health Advocates

The Professionalization of "Like Helping Like"

> *Community is as much a danger to American life as*
> *it is the foundation upon which relations are built.*
> *Community is as much a weapon in social struggles as*
> *a way to resolve such struggles. As such, it is a particu-*
> *larly effective tool for power in the United States that*
> *impinges even on those who "do not understand" the*
> *implications of the symbol.*
>
> —Hervé Varenne, "Drop in Anytime,"
> in *Symbolizing America*

"Sometimes you just have to look the other way," insisted Ron Washington to the room full of people attending a six-week training for new Community Health Advocates (CHAs). Numbering about twenty, the future outreach workers would go door-to-door in underserved neighborhoods to enroll residents as patients and clients at community agencies such as Thornton Community Health Center (TCHC), a primary care clinic that was one of three community-based organizations sponsoring the CHA program. Washington, an African American man in his fifties who had previously worked with recovering drug users, worried that people would associate the CHAs with the police if they asked too many questions. Concerned about maintaining credibility in the community, Washington felt strongly that there were some circumstances in which CHAs must not only refuse the role of state authority but also distance themselves from it by overlooking domestic violence, drug dealing, or other infractions. Others in the room, however, disagreed.

In the Freirean participatory education training for CHAs I observed in early 1998, low-income African American and Latina women and the occasional male participant were being introduced to the basics of community health outreach and prevention. Both in the training and later in their work, CHAs struggled with the boundaries of their authority and the degree to which they would be perceived as agents of the state, as articulated by Washington. Participants often worried aloud that as representatives of an agency, they would encounter suspicion from neighborhood residents. During a presentation by Carla Cisneros, a domestic violence advocate who worked for the local police department, the group considered what a CHA should do if she happened to walk into a violent domestic situation in the course of conducting outreach. Cisneros said that while "people don't usually hit each other in the presence of others," if a CHA *does* encounter this situation, it is likely an extreme one, and the best course of action is to immediately call the police. Washington objected that doing so would ruin the CHAs' credibility in the community and that they would, as a result, be seen as "narcs" ever after. Thus he felt it was better for CHAs to sometimes "look the other way." Cisneros replied that *everyone* has an ethical obligation to intervene when someone is getting hurt. She asked rhetorically, "Can I live with myself if something bad happens and I know I could have done something to prevent it?" CHAs were described as activists who organized communities for better access to health care and for greater accountability for local agencies. This dual expectation made for a central pair of contradictions: CHAs were imagined as both opponents and agents of the state and of the community they ostensibly served. Some women worried that CHAs would be seen as social workers from the Thornton Department of Social Services, widely known and feared as an agency that "took kids away" from their parents.[1]

This dilemma, of the role of CHAs in relation to the state, formed the crux of my research at TCHC. The CHA program was designed to produce community organizers who shared a vision of public health education as a technique for empowering the disenfranchised, training women on welfare to be outreach workers who would screen families for up-to-date childhood immunizations and enroll them in state-supported health insurance programs.[2]

By exploring the multiple and often contradictory demands that shape the work of CHAs, this chapter critically examines the complex relationships between the concept of community and practices of governing. I tease apart the various meanings of *community* at work within public health programs such as this to trace their effects in the governance of marginalized,

---

1. See Thompson et al. 1999 and Gilliom 1997 on welfare recipients' suspicions of surveillance by state human service agencies.
2. In an interagency collaboration initially funded by a three-year umbrella grant from the Robert Wood Johnson Foundation (RWJF), each neighborhood organization received funding through subcontracts with Healthier Communities, Inc. (HCI), the primary grant recipient. According to one program organizer, the citywide collaboration on this program was less a matter of a unified or shared vision and more an issue of political and economic expediency as multiple Thornton agencies were vying for the same funds. The differences in vision among the partner agencies only grew with time as each neighborhood agency ran into significant snags in the program and in its relationship with HCI.

urban populations. As a technology of citizenship (Cruikshank 1999), the six-week training for new CHAs mobilized the concept of community as a sign with meanings of nonprofessional authenticity (similar to street credibility), ethnic identity, and contradictory implications of marginalization and belonging. The concept of *community organizer* developed during the training posited the existence of ethnically and geographically discrete "communities" the CHAs were supposed to represent. At the same time, trainers used Freirean participatory education approaches to teach CHAs how to instantiate those communities through their community organizing around health. Through assumptions about what the term *community* refers to (e.g., culture, ethnicity, risk, poverty), community is also constituted both ideologically and pragmatically using strategies such as community mapping. Ron Washington's anxieties about being perceived as an agent of the state articulate the contradictions experienced by CHAs, who were constructed both as members of the communities they were tasked to serve and as representatives of the agencies who employed them.

In her study of meanings and uses of "community" in the construction of gay communities in San Francisco, Miranda Joseph (2002) explores communities as spaces of production and consumption. In contrast, I focus on the construction of communities as spaces of governance and difference. The CHA program highlights in vivid detail the contradictions engendered by governmental uses of the term *community* to refer to urban, poor, and/ or ethnic minority groups versus locally variable and diverse forms of identity and belonging found among groups described as "the community." The warm affective associations of the term *community* (Joseph 2002; R. Williams 1976) pull in the opposite direction from the work of categorization described by the governmental and programmatic practices discussed later. This work follows that of many scholars (e.g., Larner 2005; Marinetto 2003; Prince, Kearns, and Craig 2006; Raco, Parker, and Doak 2006) who analyze the concept of community as "an assemblage of artifacts— -political rationales, expert discourses, administrative technologies and bodies—that constitute 'its' manifold components" (Schofield 2002, 663) and extends the focus to explore an unlikely overlap between discourses of empowerment and practices of governing through community.

Meanings and Mobilization of Community in Participatory Education

I have learned the power of a reference to community. I can see through someone's use of "community" to refer to his environment. I have learned how to defend myself against a claim of community. . . . I know about true and false communities. I know how to pretend to demonstrate that I am part of a community. I believe I know how to convince people I am not pretending. I hope I can tell when my claim is legitimate. —Hervé Varenne, "Drop in Anytime," in *Symbolizing America*

Though the CHA program planners all believed strongly in the lay health advisor model (an approach with a long and proven history in public and community health; see Schoenberg et al. 2001; Eng and Young 1992; Thomas et al. 1998), program staff also recognized the need for intensive training to achieve the kinds of transformations organizers hoped for. The six-week training was based on Freirean principles of participatory education. Because it was conducted in both English and Spanish, sequential translation allowed ample time for field notes (since I was unwilling to use a recorder in the workshops). The training allowed me to observe the process of group formation among twenty or so new CHAs and to record the representations of CHAs presented therein.

The first training was held at a local community college, about fifteen minutes by car from TCHC.[3] The classroom where we met daily was filled by narrow tables arranged in a large square. Windows lined one wall, and a long erasable board was affixed to the opposite wall. Fifteen to twenty people were in the room at any given moment: mostly Puerto Rican, four to five African Americans (of these, two or three were Muslim), and one man. I was usually the only white person present. The trainers and CHA program designers—Niara Kadar, an African American Muslim with long experience in community-based organizations, and Mercedes Cota, executive director of the Latino community organization El Pueblo—were usually in the front of the room, though they stood, used the board, and circulated about the room frequently. With many participatory exercises, the training rarely took the form of straightforward lecture. A few monolingual Spanish speakers, plus several bilingual Latinos, participated in the training. To accommodate them, the first training I attended was simultaneously translated by Cota. In the second training for a new group of CHAs held a few months later, separate Spanish and English meetings were held in adjoining classrooms at the same site. Occasionally the two groups joined together for activities, but a sense of two distinct groups prevailed in the second training, despite Cota's efforts to treat them as one.

Cota and Kadar hoped to inspire CHAs through a process of consciousness-raising to serve as catalysts for their neighborhoods and continue the process of community development that began with them. CHAs' identities as "community members" were crucial to their success. The marginalized identity of African American or Latina welfare recipients became an asset to the agencies that employed them thanks to discourses of

---

3. This location seemed to introduce an additional logistical challenge for training organizers, who catered lunch each day and arranged for transportation for most of the participants, few of whom had their own transportation.

authenticity mobilized in the concept of "community." Trainers made frequent appeals to different notions of "community" when they talked about what CHAs did. The meaning of community shifted in various contexts, ranging from the strategic to the idealized to the geographic. By attending to and unpacking this range of meanings, we see that "community" was a resource that could be mobilized by multiple actors for diverse purposes. For a chronically underfunded organization such as Thornton Community Health Center, the strength and exchange value of the notion of community was its flexibility and its range of referents from the specific (e.g., to refer to the "community" of African American women in Williamsburg) to the abstract (e.g., "the black community" referring to an ethnic category).

Meanings of *community* can be roughly divided into two types—who and what is community. The term *community* sometimes describes different kinds or groups of people, such as the disenfranchised (as referred to by Freirean popular educators); members of an ethnic group; and people who are clients of agencies. Drawing on more affective connotations, *community* also refers to the sense of "common concern" noted by Raymond Williams (1976). When considering *what* community is, trainers and participants at various times drew on the affective bonds of relationship among a group of people, a force of and for collective mobilization in a community-organizing framework, or an administrative unit.

Community as "the People"

The popular education methods of Paolo Freire, Meredith Minkler, and others all rely on a notion of community that refers broadly to the disenfranchised members of a city or society. These targets of liberatory education are seen as marginalized and dependent on governmental and nongovernmental services for poor people. CHA trainers Mercedes Cota and Niara Kadar took their inspiration and pedagogical guidance from these authors and developed the CHA training following their strategies. They particularly relied on Meredith Minkler and Nina Wallerstein (1997) and others who understand public health as a practice aimed at community organizing and empowerment. As both opponents and agents of the state, health advocates were case managers of needy clients at the same time as they themselves were subject to case management by welfare. CHAs were instructed to promote agency resources to neighborhood residents but also to push for changes in the way services were provided. In practice, the identities of CHAs were shaped not only by the pedagogical efforts of the training but also through their relationships with others, including supervisors, coworkers, neighborhood residents, and other agencies. Once at work, CHAs experienced sometimes overwhelming demands on their time within these various relationships. Some community members were all too eager to take advantage of offers of help and called on CHAs for assistance with many small, unrelated tasks. Their supervisors demanded better accounting practices and more time spent in the office on paperwork and documentation. Other local agencies called on CHAs to be present for public events such as press conferences, ribbon cuttings, and the like to "represent the community" for TV cameras. The multiple demands facing CHAs rendered the simple equation made in their training, identifying them exclusively with Thornton's marginalized inner-city population, much more complex in practice.

The Contrast between "Community" and "Agencies"

The participatory education framework on which the CHA training was based sought to simultaneously educate and uplift disenfranchised groups through a process of conscientization (Freire 1974). The trainers emphasized participants' identities as "community members" as a primary focus of work in the training. Supposedly recruited to be (quasi)professionals *because* they were members of "the community," CHAs first had to learn *how* to be "community members" in a way that located them both within the target community and outside it as members of their sponsoring agencies. A series of activities were necessary to establish a particular kind of connection between CHAs and the communities they were to serve. Yet the CHAs themselves seldom spoke of "the community" until after they had completed the training. Adopting this voice of community signified their movement from part of the target population to membership in an "agency," the contrastive other to the notion of community elaborated in the training.

CHAs were called into being within a discursive framework in which community and agency were opposites, separated by a gap that needed to be filled by boundary workers who traveled back and forth between communities and agencies. Indeed, the definition of each term depended on the other. The meaning of community was often elaborated by contrasting it with its opposite, state and local agencies. *Even when minority-operated*, agencies were seen as part of a "system" that often did *not* have the best interests of "the people" at heart. Although their staff may have included individual community members, agencies nevertheless operated according to funding mandates and other administrative requirements that were impenetrable to community eyes. Agencies were gatekeepers; they had something you wanted (food stamps, food supplies, welfare benefits, free health care), so you had to do as they told you in order to get it. In the terms of this opposition, "community members" are intrinsically good, while "agencies" are possibly good but most likely difficult, unpleasant, bureaucratic, and time-consuming.

Agency staff saw community members as alienated from needed services and unwilling to engage with them. CHAs were called on to move

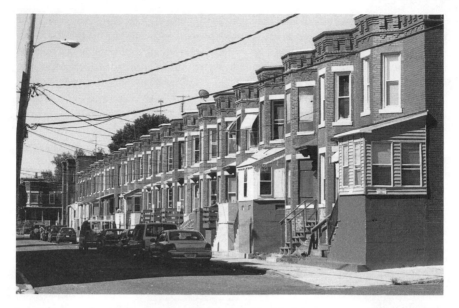

In underserved neighborhoods, Community Health Advocates went door to door to enroll residents as clients of the community-based agencies that employed them. *(Photograph courtesy of Amanda Quinby.)*

back and forth between the worlds of agency and community in order to improve access for residents of underserved neighborhoods. The opposition between "community" and "agency" could be seen in the idioms of differentiated space that characterized references to the neighborhoods where the new health advocates would do outreach. Trainers and participants alike talked about neighborhoods as being both "out there" and "in here," cut off from the professional world of service providers into which CHAs had stepped by attending this training. Neighborhoods were depicted as entire and distinct from agencies, even distant: "You go out there and talk to people" or "When we go in there, we might find. . . ."

However, the lines between "agency" and "community" were far more fluid than they first appeared. For example, both Cota and Kadar opposed the decision to pursue the Welfare-to-Work (WtW) funding that supported the program for the last six months of 1998. In one meeting in which the funding proposal was discussed, Kadar observed, "This effort was not supposed to be part of an agency [referring to yet another city agency that would lead the initiative], it's supposed to be part of the community." It is worth noting, however, that "the community" to which Kadar referred in this case was the Brighton Square Community Health Coalition, a network of service providers that she felt had greater credibility in Brighton Square than the city WtW agency.

Attributions of agency or community were racially inflected and changed in the various speech-moments in which actors were engaged. For example, Edie Anderson, a health department employee, said in a side conversation during a larger discussion about the politics of ethnic identity, "Sometimes I feel like I have a split personality" because she moved between a professional environment that was predominantly white and her black home and social life. She told me that sometimes people said she "wasn't black" because she had adapted so well to the white professional world she inhabited during the day. But she refused to accept this and reasserted her African American identity in the face of these accusations. "No, I'm black!" she said, leaning over to finish this anecdote in a whisper in my ear as the trainers sought to focus our attention back to the front of the room. Similarly, some agency staff at the training had themselves been on welfare and were able to move back and forth between positions of agency and community easily as they spoke.

How to Maintain a Community Identity That Is at Risk

CHAs were structurally positioned to negotiate, or transgress, these lines of difference. Thus they themselves served as productive sites of negotiation of the terms *agency* and *community*. TCHC's coordinator for the CHA program, Nikki Sparrow, often repeated the mantra, "We are who we serve" to her CHAs.[4] This phrase both asserted an identity between CHAs and community members and drew a distinction: CHAs are those who serve; community members are those who are served.

Pedagogically, as well, the identification of CHAs with community members was incomplete and in process. The ways that CHAs were identified with agencies or communities changed between the first and second trainings for new CHAs. In the first training Cota introduced the program by saying, "CHAs are community members who educate and serve individuals and groups to gain control over their health and their lives." A more professionalized identity for the CHA began to appear by the second training, where a handout distributed to introduce the program stated, "[CHAs are] community residents who have completed the comprehensive community health advocate certificate program to become lay outreach workers. Their mission is to bolster service coordination by forming bridges between their social networks and health and social service net-

---

4. Other authors have pointed out the contradictions that result from the multiple demands imposed on one border-spanning set of individuals. See, for example, Delamie Thompson and colleagues, who describe boundary workers also called Community Health Advocates: "CHAs may find themselves caught between program and community agendas as well as contradictions between professional and nonprofessional realms due to . . . their role as both working for the institution and being of the neighborhood" (Thompson et al. 1999, 99).

works." This change was part of a larger transformation of the training in its second iteration as it moved toward greater professionalization and sought a closer focus on more narrowly defined public health objectives.[5] For example, the "learning objectives" for the first training referred to "the importance of identity, shared values, norms, communication and helping patterns as important elements for building a sense of community." Learning objectives for the second training were more liberally sprinkled with public health terms such as *assessment* and *outcomes*. The first learning objective was rephrased as "Participants will assess the value of the CHA movement and the expected health outcomes in responding to the health concerns of children and families in [Thornton]." Similarly, while trainers emphasized their commitment to forming a "learning community" in the first training, this goal was later expressed as follows: "The purpose of this module is to introduce participants to the concepts of developing visions and missions for change in health status of communities by looking at healthy environments and resources in neighborhoods for children." Even before the program received WtW funding described in Chapter 3, changes between the first and second CHA trainings reflected pressure to rearticulate the program's goals in terms that were more compatible with the public health emphasis on professionalization and measurable effectiveness (see Gupta and Sharma 2006, 288–289).

Insofar as CHAs were called on to traverse the gap between "the community" and "agencies," CHAs' identities *as* members of the community were seen as crucial to their credibility and legitimacy. The CHAs were Puerto Rican or African American women, as were most of the residents who would later take advantage of their services. Shared ethnic identities were sometimes glossed as "looking like" the people to whom the CHAs did outreach. Resemblance was also figured as "membership" in a common "community," understood as a social network as well as similar habits, speech, and style. This kind of resemblance served as an entry pass into what were often called, in public-health-speak, "hard to reach" neighborhoods or populations.[6] In a very segregated city in which suspicion of outsiders was ingrained, simply "looking like" those whose doors one knocked on was believed to facilitate entry and acceptance. CHAs were assumed to have shared experiences with the people in the "target" neighborhoods and were instructed to draw on their experiences of raising children and coping with poverty as they went door-to-door talking with mothers about their kids' health. Shared experience was supposed to not

5. See Pigg 2001 for a discussion of the didactic nature of biomedical and public health "trainings" that situates them within broader contexts of language and modernity.
6. Joel Meister and colleagues turn this notion of "hard to reach" on its head by calling the lay health workers in a prenatal outreach program "hard to reach" when they showed increasing interest in spending more time in the office rather than doing outreach to clients' homes (Meister et al. 1992, 45).

only allow entrée and build rapport but also give CHAs increased credibility among other low-income women of color. The idea of "speaking the
same language," literally and figuratively, came up often in conversations
about outreach. Habits of speech, bodily style, "street smarts"—all were
believed to function even more effectively than the ID cards CHAs wore in
gaining them access to people's homes.

Once the CHAs' expertise as community members was recruited and
mobilized, however, it was jeopardized as they came to identify with the
health center and the professional expertise it represented. The CHAs felt
ambivalent about the seductions offered by this professional world. For
many CHAs, this was the first time they had worked in the compara-
tively "white collar" environment of the health center. Because they were
enrolled in a welfare training program, they also received free day care and
bus tokens to pay for their transportation to and from work. They took
full advantage of the access to telephones and fax and copy machines they
found at the clinic. As others have described in greater detail (Finn and
Underwood 2000), maintaining welfare and other benefits such as food
stamps requires constant communication and "verification" with state
social workers. CHAs were delighted to be able, some for the first time, to
fax this paperwork to their caseworkers. They stood at the copy machine
photocopying immunization records, pay stubs, or tax forms with the busy
officiousness of underpaid, overworked bureaucrats.

At the same time, CHAs were also admonished to maintain their
community identification in order to reach so-called hard-to-reach populations—a phrase that points to the separation between community members and agencies. A health education guest lecturer cautioned the CHAs,
"Never forget where you came from. When we separate ourselves from
the people we serve, we can't be effective." Her emphasis on maintaining an identification with "the community" seemed to call for an almost
intentional resistance against these professionalizing tendencies. Thus even
agency staff acknowledged that the layering of professional experiences on
top of community experience helps form new subjectivities for people in
this position.[7]

CHAs' position "in between" agency and community worked against
any simple identity between CHAs and "community." The work of providing help to families seemed to introduce a distance between the health
advocates and community members. Beyond enrolling people into a primary health care center and assisting them with Medicaid applications,

---

7. For an outline of a parallel case that explores racialized echoes of the construction of
difference in Dutch colonialism, see Li 2007. This work gives a careful analysis of the
ways in which Dutch colonists engaged in the "creative (re)construction" of "the native-
ness of Native" Indonesians "to restore Natives to their authentic state" following colonial
contact (46).

CHAs also carried a vast mandate to provide "any other help you might need" through information and referrals. This thrust the CHA into a social worker–like helping position as she negotiated between community members and agencies by making referrals and following up on them. The language CHAs used to describe their work revealed how they were pulled between different models of friendship, social work, and pastoral assistance. CHAs would use the word *clients* in a troubled[8] way to refer to the people they helped. Occasionally a CHA would refer to "my client," but more often she would say "my little old lady," "my seventeen-year-old girl," or "that guy I met on the street," or refer to a person by name. These verbal cues indicated the CHAs' ambivalence about understanding themselves as social workers when their position as welfare recipients likely gave them many compelling reasons *not* to identify with that particular subject-position.

Some CHAs saw their work in terms that were framed by their church experiences, evoking an ecumenical context as they talked about "helping" people "less fortunate" than themselves. Others saw the process of establishing trusting relationships with neighborhood residents as befriending individuals or families. However, this kind of relationship also caused a certain stress if a CHA felt ethically obligated to act in a direction she was unable to fully pursue. Maebelle Tye described her dilemma about a particular family of whom she was quite fond:

> My problem with that family [is that] I'm not able to keep that [*pauses, grasping for the right word*] contact? Because they brought me in as a stranger. . . . I had never met them before, just knocking on their door. . . . They made me feel comfortable, but I haven't been able to follow up with them. I made the son an appointment; he canceled that appointment, so I went back and I talked with them like I would with *my* brother or family member. I said, "Look, if you can't make that appointment, what time would you like to be there? They close at a certain time on Monday. You wanted that appointment at five o'clock; I was able to work it at five o'clock." Okay. He came to that one. But I haven't been able to find out how the appointment went, you know, what happened.

The conduct of CHAs as representatives of publicly funded NGOs in relation to neighborhood residents was an ethical question. For example, when someone asked in the training if CHAs were mandated reporters of child abuse according to state law, Kadar seemed to feel that if community members are not clients of CHAs, neither are CHAs mandated reporters. But since this was a gray area, it turned into a conversation

---

8. See Judith Butler's sense of the word (Butler 1990).

about what the ethical obligations of CHAs were, to whom, under what circumstances. Specific categories of care providers (medical staff, school staff, social workers) are required by state law to report suspected incidents of child abuse to the department of social services. As concerned community members, CHAs would want to intervene on the child's behalf if they suspected or encountered child abuse. However, few CHAs would have been comfortable actually making a report to the department of social services because of the poor reputation of that agency in the community. The health advocates had a difficult time articulating themselves into positions of governmental responsibility, even while they were called upon to assume that role both by their job descriptions and by their personal sense of ethical obligation.[9] CHAs' struggles to both shed and maintain their identities as community members echo new formations of expertise generated in neoliberal approaches to governing that dislocate expertise from its traditional moorings (Epstein 1996) while opening it to contestation (a process I explore further in another health care domain in Chapter 4). In an examination of public-private community development partnership, Wendy Larner uncovers the emergence of heterogeneous conceptions of community and emphasizes "the new spaces, socialities and subjectivities of social policy, including . . . the rise of community-based expertise" associated with the devolution of funds, responsibility, and programs to the local, nongovernmental level (2005, 13). Understanding CHAs as agents of government helps us consider the kinds of changes in the way government happens now and the reformulations of subjectivity that accompany neoliberal governance (Joseph 2002, 74).

The Depoliticized Discourse of "Community"

In addition to using the term *community* to contrast laypeople or clients with agencies and their staff, many public health workers I met used the word *community* to refer to people of color or to cultural difference in general. For instance, "Your agency doesn't have enough *community* representation" might be a charge leveled against an organization with an all-white board of directors.[10] However, I seldom heard participants use this term to describe themselves or other people of color unless they had already spent some time working in social services. They were much more likely to refer to various groups by name—"Latinos," "Puerto Ricans," "blacks," or "black folks"—or to use notions of *family* or *neighborhood*

9. See also Gupta and Sharma 2006 on outreach workers' identification with and refusal of state roles in an empowerment program for women in India (286, 290).
10. See similar charges discussed in Chapter 4, at a 2008 conference in which attendees at a workshop sponsored by the Joint Commission brainstormed criteria that surveyors might use to evaluate hospitals and health care organizations on their adherence to norms of culturally appropriate health care.

to describe the structures of identification that helped locate them in a particular social milieu and in geographic space. Cota and Kadar frequently mentioned the importance of the political representation of people of color (in their words), both in city politics and in community-based organizations such as Helping the Black Family. Similarly, Miranda Joseph, in her study of community-based organizations serving San Francisco's lesbian and gay community, shows how "nonprofits often stand for community metonymically. . . . [N]onprofits are asked to represent communities politically, to speak for the communities for which they are metonyms" (Joseph 2002, 70).[11] Agencies in Thornton seemed to struggle with the expectation to appear "community-based," defined by the direct participation of "community members" in agency governance (see Chapter 3 for an extended consideration of the concept of "community participation"). For example, Cota often mentioned Doña Anir, an elderly member of El Pueblo's community advisory board, and the active voice she had in the priorities of the organization.

Part of what the language of community does is to allow agencies and program administrators to refer to racial or ethnic groups without mentioning them as such. Staff members from the Thornton Health Department often used *community* to refer to people of color, and specifically to African Americans in Thornton. It hosted annual "community speakouts" called Community Voices Addressing Infant Mortality. The event I attended with the CHAs had an invited list of many minority organizations. It was clear that the "community" both at risk and in question was the African American community, particularly the low-income black neighborhoods in which high infant mortality rates clustered. Referring to a "community" instead of an ethnic group works to depoliticize claims that are in truth made on behalf of particular ethnic groups. Community thus functions as a "third way" of government that is seen as less political and more naturally valued and positive (Joseph 2002; Larner 2005; Prince, Kearns, and Craig 2006). Throughout this book, I seek to subject the naturalizing claims of community (Gupta and Ferguson 1997), like those of ethnicity and public health, to critical analysis to identify the uses to which these concepts are put and their wide-ranging capacities and effects.

Like categorical uses of the term *community* to refer to certain ethnic groups without explicitly mentioning ethnicity, the medically underserved neighborhood in which TCHC was located was another frequently used statistical and bureaucratic designation (which TCHC's first executive

---

11. David Harvey, in his *Brief History of Neoliberalism*, observes that while NGOs have emerged as a key tool of governance under neoliberalism, theirs is an ambivalent practice of representation: "[NGOs] often control their clientele rather than represent it. They claim and presume to speak on behalf of those who cannot speak for themselves, even define the interests of those they speak for. . . . But the legitimacy of their status is always open to doubt" (2005, 177).

director had a hand in establishing; see Shaw 2005). Within that medically underserved area, each CHA was responsible, as described shortly, for specific "target neighborhoods."[12] Statistical representations of a population, such as the percentage of poor people in a certain neighborhood, are always simplifications produced for particular purposes. Anthropologist James Scott points out that states make these abstracted representations to serve a limited number of ends. He writes:

> No administrative system is capable of representing any existing social community except through a heroic and greatly schematized process of abstraction and simplification. It is not simply a question of capacity, although, like a forest, a human community is surely far too complicated and variable to easily yield its secrets to bureaucratic formulae. It is also a question of purpose. State agents have no interest . . . in describing an entire social reality. . . . Their abstractions and simplifications are disciplined by a small number of objectives. (1998, 23)

The health advocates themselves were identified through similar practices of categorization: they were poor, welfare mothers, African Americans, or Puerto Ricans; these categorizations, as we will see in the following chapter, soon became even narrower and more specific, focusing on levels of education, substance abuse, and individual work histories. Each designation placed the CHA as a member of a population, classifications that were not only reductive but also productive of certain subject-positions or possible identifications.

"You Gotta Do a Little Analysis": Creating Communities through Organizing

Trainers taught that community, in its affective, relational sense, was also created through community organizing. Cota and Kadar led the participants through exercises designed to represent the practice of community organizing on a small scale. Community organizing is a method to improve health in disenfranchised populations by increasing their control over their health (Braithwaite, Bianchi, and Taylor 1994; Minkler and Wallerstein 1997). Community organizing projects often rely on participatory education techniques as an empowerment tool. In this method, community members come together to identify problems and take action for their

---

12. The linguistic construction "target neighborhood" or "target community" reveals the directionality and power dynamics inherent in this kind of health promotion program. See Fischer and Poland 1998.

solution. Participatory education emphasizes the importance of lived experience and knowledge of the people who are being educated. For example, at the beginning of each training Cota and Kadar distributed a list of "assumptions of the training": the belief that "communities can solve their own problems; . . . resources can be found at a local level; . . . the entire community must be involved; . . . [and solutions should] build on existing experience and expertise." This was also described as an assets-mapping approach (Turner, McKnight, and Kretzmann 1999), as a counter to conventional public health "needs assessments" that focus on a community's weaknesses rather than its strengths.

Freirean approaches to adult education, widely used both in the United States and in international development efforts, are supposed to contravene the hierarchical power arrangements implicit in traditional education and to produce empowered "learners" (Gupta and Sharma 2006). Cota described empowerment as the ability "to find out what is going on in the community, engage in a process to allow the people to gain control of the problems that are going on in their life, to get them to experience their power."[13] For the trainers, "education is never neutral, it always has a goal, perspective, or objective"—in this case, helping new health advocates generate an "analysis of oppression." Individual empowerment seemed to depend on the health advocates developing this analysis. Its key components included an understanding of social identity; class, the distribution of wealth and access to health care; and community organizing and education techniques for CHAs. This analysis was supposed to drive the CHAs' interactions with community members and their understanding of the larger public health picture of Thornton. As community organizers, CHAs were supposed to carry, mobilize, and extend this analysis in their work with other neighborhood residents. Kadar summed up their philosophy by saying, "Here's what you have to keep in mind in your work. People are dealing with circumstances that are difficult sometimes. If the information you're bringing isn't related to people's lives, don't give it to them. It isn't about just going in and telling someone, 'I'm going to teach you about this issue.' You gotta do a little analysis."

The implicit designation of CHAs' work, particularly the elements associated with community uplift, as women's work echoes the gendered distribution of work in community development projects elsewhere. Anthropologist Kate Crehan studied an arts-based project in an East London housing project that was organized and carried out by women, following a similar logic. Crehan observes, "Often, it seems, the work that goes into making 'the community' a more pleasant place to live, which frequently involves a lot of unpaid voluntary labor, is seen as somehow the responsibility of women, part of their maternal role as 'homemakers.' It

13. The concept of empowerment is discussed in further detail in Chapter 3.

is noteworthy that on many of the estates on which Free Form [the arts organization she studied] has worked, the key activists among the tenants have been women" (2006, 61; see also Goode 2001, 372).

Building on these expectations, the kind of ideal citizen being formed in this training was a change agent who works for community empowerment around health (see also, e.g., Gastaldo 1997). CHAs were supposed to replicate the process of empowerment that they experienced in the training in the work they did in target neighborhoods. Once the health advocates started work, however, their work was constrained by more prosaic, categorical considerations described in detail in the following chapter. They found themselves confronted by agency contracts that obligated them to report a certain number of "contacts" every week, or to process a certain number of Medicaid enrollments per month. Like the outreach workers described by Aradhana Sharma (Gupta and Sharma 2006), the health advocates expressed frustration with "getting the numbers" when they compared this kind of work with the mission of community organizing for social change that had been described to them in the training. The contrast between different models of citizenship that operated in the training and in the "real world" seemed paradoxically to work against their engagement in the larger issues of community uplift presented in the training. While Cota and Kadar worked to produce model citizens who exemplified ideals of community commitment and a structural understanding of injustice, the actual work assigned to CHAs fostered instead a notion of citizenship as being a productive worker, with greater emphasis on meeting contract obligations and producing measurable outcomes.

The community organization work by health advocates would, according to this model, result in the emergence of a community as a political subject, a process that was facilitated by women's roles as providers of pragmatic assistance.[14] By going door to door and talking with families, CHAs were supposed to serve as a literal vehicle of communication to help this emergent community identify its health needs. In their dual role as both agency staff and community representatives, health advocates would relay information about community needs back to agencies to help facilitate solutions. This carrying back and forth of information would

---

14. A similar kind of emergent understanding of community, tied to practices of community organizing, is described by Kate Crehan, who studied a community arts program in Provost, a public housing estate in East London. She concludes, "The key point, I would suggest, is that there was *not* some preexisting Provost 'community' with which it was Free Form's [the arts organization] task to connect. Rather there was a multitude of both social networks and narratives of identity and belonging that different people might or might not claim. . . . The Free Form project can be seen as providing a space in which it was possible—but by no means inevitable—for a particular sense of community to emerge" (2006, 73; emphasis added). See also Larner 2005 on the differences between the geographically and ethnically defined communities that emerged from a New Zealand community development program, with particular attention to the exclusions entailed in each.

contribute to the formation of a social body, one that was bounded by geography and ethnicity and instantiated by women's gendered roles as communicators. This idea of community was organized according to the community-agency dichotomy described earlier. It would be constituted by its members' common "needs," but those needs were implicitly defined in relation to the services (including the health advocates themselves) of local agencies. The emergence of this community with shared needs and a common voice, embodied in the CHA, can be said to be a political subject insofar as it would then participate in dialogue on a local level. On a broader level, Pierre Bourdieu draws our attention to the power of social movement leaders who actualize an entity where one previously did not exist, by means of both acting upon and embodying the "common sense" of a population:

> The capacity for bringing into existence in an explicit state, . . . of making public (i.e., objectified, visible, sayable, and even official) that which, not yet having attained objective and collective existence, remained in a state of individual or serial existence—people's disquiet, anxiety, expectation, worry [or needs]—represents a formidable social power, that of bringing into existence groups by establishing the common sense, the explicit consensus, of the whole group. (1991, 236)

In community health, discourses of health disparities help articulate the "common sense" understanding of a bounded, contiguous and unitary "community" with common health needs. Fostering that shared vision was part of the job of the CHA.

Participants in the CHA training seemed to share this sense of homology between the individual and community transformation. For example, in reviewing a day's activities, Viviana said, "I learned that one voice can make a difference. I saw Mercedes stand up there with one voice, and she touched all of us, and now there are thirteen voices and we can make some noise." Community organizing is the process of producing or imposing meaning on groups of people. A "community" can be seen, in Bourdieu's terms, as a theoretical class. Community organizing performs the labor of categorization by establishing a group or people or a neighborhood as a "community." By relaying information, holding community events, and relying on case studies to convey their analyses, community organizers and trainers make interventions in the field of cultural production and create objectified representations of the social world (Bourdieu 1991, 236–237).

Thus, an important meaning of "community" as used by trainers was a force of and for collective mobilization. Kadar illustrated this concept of community with the example of a hanging mobile, drawing it on the board. She reminded people that individual community members are resources to be used, and that they have connections to other community members, just as when you move one piece of a mobile, every other piece moves. This notion of collective mobilization was echoed in definitions of *community* offered by participants in one exercise. When asked to define *community*, people mentioned coming together, a "common cause," and cooperation ("people who live in peace, who get together to help each other"), while others mentioned unity and safety. Similarly, on their applications for the CHA program, prospective participants answered questions including, "When you hear the word *community* what do you think?" In their written responses, women tended to mention relationships ("togetherness"), mutual aid, and geography, for example, "working for the people in the area; people who sometimes need help; many people living in a certain area; helping people around that are in need." When asked, "What do you consider to be a healthy community?" one woman wrote, "I consider a community being healthy when they bond together as one." Some described notions of security and hygiene: safety seemed to mean specifically "a drug-free environment" or "gang-free."

While communities are clearly instantiated or brought into existence by this kind of organizing, some sense of connection between individuals nevertheless seems to exist before the act of organizing. Kadar recognized this when participants in the first training had no difficulty listing a variety of positive characteristics of Thornton, in an exercise that asked participants to describe Thornton to an outsider. She said, "It's already there, the community we want to build." And yet the authenticity of community is also, like the community identity of CHAs, always in doubt. With a nod to the normative value of community as an unattainable ideal, Hervé Varenne describes an understanding of community as always at risk, always in doubt: "[Those who perform community] must doubt that they have achieved community, if only because someone will always doubt their sincerity" (1986, 226). Poststructuralist theories of subjectivity further destabilize concepts of community by unlinking identity from its naturalized moorings. As Miranda Joseph notes, "Foucauldian theories of the subject as an unstable effect of discourse rather than an authentic origin of identity suggested that there was not unity within the individual subject, let alone members of a community, and put into doubt the authorizing and naturalizing origin stories on which community formation so often depends" (2002, xxv). The effort to translate individual CHAs' experiences into the structural insights CHA trainers hoped would foster a sense of community as constituted by shared ethnic identity and experiences of oppression were not always successful. These failures of translation occurred both in cases of linguistic translation from English to Spanish in the CHA training and in conceptual moments wherein trainers sought to help participants reinterpret their experiences in terms of their "analysis of oppression."

Translating Experience, or the Limits
of Mobilizing Community

Sherry Simon (1990) points out two different purposes of linguistic translation—translation that seeks to *replace* the original with an equivalent text not identifiable as "foreign," and *supplemental* translation, which carries "something additional," some cultural weight from the original. Simultaneous translation between English and Spanish in both trainings met this latter goal of supplemental translation, insofar as Cota clearly felt that bringing different language groups together as one served goals other than function or efficiency. Simultaneous translation meant that someone would make a comment, or a brief exchange would take place, and Cota would nod and hold up a finger to pause further conversation while she translated the comment, whether English or Spanish. Over time, her translation became part of the conversation itself, as she repeated comments yet moved the conversation forward in an iterative process. By holding bilingual English and Spanish trainings, Cota and Kadar initially tried to prefigure the cohesive yet multicultural society that CHAs were supposed to help build. Despite this intent, considerations of efficiency superseded their prefigurative goals, and the second training was primarily monolingual, held in two groups with only occasional joint, bilingual sessions.

Cota served as translator so consistently that she became identified with that role to the exclusion of anyone else. Even participants who were fully bilingual occasionally relied on her for translation even though they could have translated their own comments. Cota frequently referred to her Chicana background and seemed to embody the figure of mediator between different groups—she was not Anglo or African American or Puerto Rican, but she could relate to aspects of each.[15] As translator, Cota was a passage point through which most conversation traveled. By translating, Cota authorized participants' words, especially when she commented on their comments—"very important point; let me translate that"—before she did so. She excelled at the process of "active listening," reflecting people's comments back to them *before* she translated and thanking them for their contribution.

When the Spanish and English groups did come together for activities in the second, monolingual training, a sense of overall group cohesiveness was slower in emerging than in the previous training, where people were more likely to cross lines of linguistic or ethnic difference around such casual issues as sharing a cigarette, a ride, or a meal. Returning to the practice of simultaneous translation in this larger combined group, Cota's translation seemed clunky, awkward, and repetitive instead of effortless, an interruption in the day's usual events. In the first training I observed,

---

15. See Simon 1996 (ch. 2) on the figure of the translator as cultural mediator.

her translation was integrated into the fabric of the training (for example, everything was printed in English and Spanish) and became almost invisible because it was habitual. Now people became more obviously restless and fidgety when Cota paused to translate something.

There were other times when translation failed, despite Cota's efforts. For example, during a conversation about the "American Dream" (described as owning a house, car, etc.), Iris Molino told a story about getting fired because a criminal background check revealed her history of drug use. Iris told this story in English and commented that this experience taught her that she was excluded from attaining the American Dream because she had been arrested for using drugs. When she finished her story, Cota commented, "This is a very important point; let me translate that" into Spanish—when Iris, who was comfortably bilingual, could have easily translated for herself. *Mid-translation*, however, Cota switched back to English to describe the legal "standards" that Iris failed to meet in her employment. With her English-speaking co-trainer, as well, Cota would occasionally interrupt to translate and then end up rephrasing Kadar's point *in English*, without always back-translating into Spanish again. The same thing happened with Spanish speakers: when a bilingual woman commented in Spanish that racial stereotyping and prejudice kept children from reaching their potential, Cota said again, "Good point," and began to translate this into English, but when she reached the crux of the point ("the child's potential is not allowed to flower"), she switched back to Spanish. Conversations about the U.S. judicial system or legal requirements seemed to require English, perhaps as articulations of national identity that somehow defy translation.[16]

Other kinds of translation took place during the first, bilingual training in addition to linguistic translation. CHA trainers were actively involved in what Freire calls the process of conscientization, as part of their work on CHAs' identities. In both CHA trainings I observed, Cota and Kadar sought to translate the details of participants' everyday lives into more structurally oriented generalizations and analyses in the process of participatory education. For example, conscientization entailed first helping participants perceive social hierarchies and their places within them, before giving them the "tools" to change the hierarchies through collective action. Kadar said once, "There's a social identity you are born into, that you are stuck with." Social identity was also defined as "the ways that people perceive us. . . . It's going to affect your life." Practices of translation

---

16. Stacy Pigg (2001) analyzes the ways in which certain kinds of knowledge and information seem to require English terminology in AIDS education efforts in Nepal. Further research may consider what aspects of government in the United States likewise depend on English for communication.

highlighted the lack of connection between the trainers' goals—to produce a certain kind of subject (community organizer)—and the participants' experiences. Translation practices also pointed to larger determinants that shaped the training (e.g., English dominance) despite trainers' efforts to keep the process egalitarian and participatory.

Trainers engaged participants in a process of ethical reflection (Geary 2007), in which trainers tried to help the new health advocates reinterpret their own lives in terms of this analysis. Cota commented, "It's important for CHAs to do an analysis in our communities. This means we must ask *why*, for example, there are such high rates of AIDS in our communities. We can't just have little programs, we have to have an analysis of why we have these problems." To foster this analysis of the structural causes of poverty and other issues, trainers distributed page-long "case studies" from actual events to illustrate concepts of hegemony, discrimination, racism, privilege, and so on and presented them to the group for discussion. These case studies met with mixed success; while trainers were trying to translate CHAs' everyday lives into broader, structural insights, the new health advocates generally maintained a focus on the details of their lived experience. The case study was intended to provide the group a concrete example to which they could relate, but its purpose was to bring them to more general insights about the nature of oppression in society. The case study here functioned as a political tool, but its limitation was in its specificity—the health advocates would, in response, share details of *their* everyday lives that corresponded to the case study, while not necessarily articulating the "take-home points" that the trainers had in mind. For example, a case study about a slumlord whose building caught fire generated multiple stories from participants about various slumlords they had known, but few specific suggestions of the kind the trainers were looking for about possible actions the hypothetical residents could take to obtain adequate housing or hold the landlord accountable. From moments like this, then, it was unclear how successful the participatory education method was in translating participants' lives into more abstract levels of insight.

These examples illustrate the difficulties encountered by participatory education practitioners who seek to "empower" women on welfare through this technology of citizenship. Translation practices in the first training did allow Hispanic, African American, and other participants to share dialogue and engage with each other around common issues presented by the trainers. However, when expediency forced the separation of English and Spanish speakers into two groups on a daily basis, occasional simultaneous translation was inadequate to meet the goal of cultivating connections between different participants. Finally, participatory education techniques were not always adequate to achieve translation of participants' everyday lives into the kinds of structural analyses fostered by the trainers.

Lay Health Advisors: Knowing and Governing the Poor

During the 19th century, private organizations bore much of the burden of support for dependency. Unpaid laymen, equipped with the desire to do good and with the compelling urge to shape the value system of the poor, mobilized important philanthropic resources. —Oscar Handlin, "Foreword," in Lubove, *The Professional Altruist*

So we know that from a medical point of view [and] from a population perspective, finding illness long after it's proceeded to the point where it's manifest is way off base if we're going to measure a whole community. —Philip Weaver, M.D., founder of the Brighton Square CHA program

The practice of relying on low-income women to deliver information to their peers in the hope of encouraging greater use of health services and to contribute to the development of the community has a long history. A community health center in Pholela, South Africa, in the early 1950s is often cited as the first example of community health workers (CHWs) doing health education using a population-based model (Kark and Kark 1999; Tollman 1994). Pholela community health workers were each responsible for twenty-five to thirty homes in an "initial defined area" (Tollman 1994, 654). CHWs provided health education, gathered data on families, and "coordinated care of individuals with interventions directed toward changing health-related behavior of families and the community" (Tollman 1994, 654). In the United States, lay health advisors gained popularity in the 1960s and 1970s as a way to address the perceived social distance between health care providers and the communities they served (Eng and Young 1992). The model was adapted from international health and development organizations that used laypeople, often women, to promote development programs in the global South (Wellin 1955).

Public health and other literature cites lack of trust or respect as an important deterrent to the utilization of health care and other services by poor people and people of color in the United States. Lay health advisors were supposed to be a more effective vehicle for health information and recruitment than other health professionals, who were seen as separated from the people they served by barriers of culture and class (Earp et al. 1997; Eng and Young 1992; Salber 1979). Residential and social segregation have historically contributed to the perceived need for minority health care providers to serve minorities who were unable to receive care from white health care providers. As Keith Wailoo (2001) eloquently shows in his history of African American health care in Memphis, Tennessee, when segregation mandates separation of white health care providers from black patients, black health care providers are then called on to traverse legally and socially separate worlds. Outreach workers and lay health advisors are similar kinds of boundary workers, albeit with less professional credentialing than the minority health care providers Wailoo studies. In fact, their lack of advanced training *obscures* the professional-client relationship between CHAs and neighborhood residents in a way that CHAs at times found quite confusing.

The lay health worker model grew out of a strong belief in the efficacy of "like helping like." "Friendly visitors," for example, were a feature of "charity organization societies" in Victorian England as well as in the United States. Friendly visitors represented a new model of helping the poor, what advocates called "scientific charity," because of the role home visitors played in gathering information and "diagnosing" the problems of needy families. "Not alms, but a friend" was the motto of Boston Associated Charities in the 1880s (Lubove 1965), as philanthropists tried to devise a new method in which informal and affective relationships between middle-class women and the poor supplanted the patronizing relations of alms. Home visitors lent aid and support, but rarely financial relief, to the worthy struggling poor. Then as now, it was thought that direct charity, or alms, contributed to the "dependency" of the poor, while "work was a universal panacea for problem families" (Lubove 1965, 8). Friendly visitors enacted gendered norms of caregiving, formalizing and regularizing existing norms of support among women and transferring them across class boundaries.

Home visits sought to enlist the participation of the poor in their own uplift, to help them see their character flaws and bad judgment that needed to change if they were to help themselves out of poverty (Cruikshank 1999). It was the special skill of the home visitor to be able to diagnose the particular flaws challenging each family and to aid in its "treatment." Lay health advisor programs and contemporary welfare reform share a mission to "work on" the character of the poor (Rosenberg 1987) by encouraging them to be active, involved community members (as described here) or productive citizens (as in Chapter 3). Both the CHA program and its predecessors functioned as "technologies of government" (Dean 1999), practical forms of intervention that first specified populations and then sought to influence their behavior and subjectivities (Pigg 2001).

Proxy and Portrait: Practices of Representation through Community Mapping

According to Dr. Philip Weaver, a primary care physician who was a principal architect of the CHA program in Brighton Square, the difficulty in funding programs that provide preventive health care for poor communities is their inability to demonstrate their effectiveness on a *population-wide* level, through indexes such as increased health care utilization or decreased diabetes rates or emergency room utilization. Too many factors influence health and health care utilization, Weaver argued, for any single program to be able to show change on a large scale. Instead, he proposed *narrowing the population* in question to a radius of a few square blocks.[17] If a health organization could mark off a hundred-square-block area and make sure that every family within it had health insurance and quality, culturally appropriate health care, the health status of those families would demonstrably improve. The CHA program emerged in part as an answer to this vision. In cooperation with a group of service providers in one neighborhood of Thornton, he developed a coordinated outreach program to serve this purpose. He divided the neighborhood into zones and designated an outreach worker for each zone, each with three hundred families under her purview. Each outreach worker would be familiar with all important neighborhood programs. They would conduct an assessment of each family's "needs" and make referrals to local programs. It was a locally based system of coordinated care developed to track and show change in one population's health status: community health as accounting method, and as technology of government, at the neighborhood level. CHAs used community maps and door-to-door outreach to create access to populations that were previously designated "hard to reach" or "hard to serve." Based on the maps, CHAs were assigned to zones of, for example, five square blocks, and they were responsible for meeting the needs of all the families who lived in their zone. These zones were created according to the reduced scale cited by Weaver earlier, which would allow them to show an actual change in the health status of residents of those zones. In this way CHAs serve as agents of governance of populations not previously accessible to service providers or government.

This community outreach approach opens neighborhoods to intervention and scrutiny in new ways, at the same time that CHAs undoubtedly did bring help to some families who needed it—accessible, low-cost health care to people who lacked it, for example. And as active subjects constructing their own professional identities, CHAs often administered the program as they saw fit, accommodating a family's needs in a more flexible way than typical social service programs. Nonetheless, as discussed further shortly, CHAs, as women on welfare themselves, were also subject to neoliberal rationalities when they began to participate in this WtW program. Population-based health care is thus a tool for surveillance and control as much as for the delivery of services and expanding access.

---

17. The Harlem Children's Zone (Spielman et al. 2006; Nicholas et al. 2005; Tough 2004) is a related initiative that proposed to address disparities in education, achievement, and income in one New York City neighborhood by similarly narrowing the field of intervention to a sixty-square-block radius and intensively intervening on a population-wide level with all residents in that area.

Mapping and Governing Communities

One of the ways communities were constituted was by means of representations created by a technique known as *community mapping*. For their first "field assignment" for the CHA training, participants returned to their home neighborhoods and drew in detail their immediate surroundings. The field assignment instructed them to "map your community within four blocks of your home, street by street. Draw out the housing, stores, lots, schools, etc." The community mapping technique had two conceptual foundations in public health, "population-based health care," outlined earlier, and assets mapping (Kretzmann and McKnight 1993). The mapping of communities had the important effect of making "hard to reach" neighborhoods legible, accessible and subject to the state's power via the CHAs. As Nikolas Rose describes, "The government of a population . . . becomes possible only through discursive mechanisms that represent the domain to be governed as an intelligible field with specifiable limits and particular characteristics. . . . This is a matter of defining boundaries, rendering that within them visible, assembling information about that which is included and devising techniques to mobilize the forces and entities thus revealed" (1999, 33). Dr. Philip Weaver, member of the Brighton Square Community Health Coalition, described the population-based health care approach to me in an interview. Each CHA would be responsible for identifying and tracking every household and family within her assigned zone. She would make successive home visits to first determine the number of adults and children therein, the immunization status of each child in the household, the insurance status of each member, and so on.[18] Her subsequent intervention with a family was determined by what needs she found: those lacking health insurance received assistance with a Medicaid application; those needing a primary care provider were referred to the health center; those who were food insecure were given food stamp applications.

As they visually surveyed their "zones" and created their own representations of the populations, structures, and resources within them, CHAs began to *constitute* the communities they were supposed to organize. Identifying families and assessing needs was a means by which CHAs organized communities according to geography. In the process, the empowerment model constituted "communities" as political subjects with needs, rights, and a "voice" projected through the CHA. At the same time, through community mapping, communities became terrains of government, or communities of intervention, a way of transferring

---

18. Julie Brownlie and Alexandra Howson show how negotiations between doctors and patients in Scotland about immunizations are an integral part of "governing health at a distance" as immunization adherence is an "obligatory . . . part of 'good citizenship'" (2006, 433).

the responsibility of government to local or sublocal groups. Instead of relying on federal or state government to provide accessible health care or full employment, these local groups such as TCHC or the Brighton Square Community Health Coalition now become responsible, through the mechanism of the CHA program, for maintaining a proper relationship to health.

The constituting of communities also opens them for intervention by agents such as CHAs, social workers, or other health workers. As noted by anthropologist and political scientist James Scott (1998) in another context, "These state simplifications [here, the neighborhood maps made by CHAs] . . . were maps that, when allied with state power, would enable much of the reality they depicted to be remade" (3). The state power here is the CHAs, working for TCHC, a federally funded clinic, and two other community organizations. Community agencies, as agents of the state, wish to remake these "target communities" in various ways: those still motivated by a desire for community empowerment envision communities in which residents are not only employed but also politically organized and active—they vote, they are civic-minded, and they talk with each other about what is good for "the community." On the other hand, those motivated by a belief in the bootstrapping mentality of WtW (described in the following chapter) envision a community in which children are raised by two-parent families in which mothers stay home to raise the kids—or, barring that, single-parent families in which mothers work in order to provide financial support and a good role model for their children. In other words, partly as a response to the devolution of federal services to a local level, and partly because organizations are created as change-making institutions, community agencies regardless of their position on the political spectrum practice techniques of government.

As a designer of the CHA program, Philip Weaver believed that the program's ultimate aim was to improve the health of designated populations in each of the three target neighborhoods. Before he became involved with the CHA program, Weaver had spearheaded the institutionalization of the Brighton Square Community Health Coalition, a group of health care and other service providers, to coordinate services and outreach efforts for that neighborhood.[19] Weaver felt that the Brighton Square neighborhood was especially appropriate for implementing a population-based approach to primary health care because it was a small neighborhood with clearly demarcated geographic boundaries provided by a river, a highway,

---

19. Despite, or perhaps because of, its poverty, Brighton Square suffered no lack of social and other services, and providers often complained of stepping on each other's toes in the relatively small territory. Weaver brought together Fielding Hospital, El Pueblo, the neighborhood councils, and other smaller organizations with the promise of better community participation in their programs through coordinated outreach efforts.

and tracts of industrial sprawl. Brighton Square was ethnically homogeneous and mostly low-income. A population that was 90 percent Puerto Rican meant fewer language barriers for outreach workers to overcome. Weaver also attributed the program's success to a stable population and a greater degree of social connections among residents than in some other Thornton neighborhoods.

Weaver felt strongly that health care had to be "facilitated" because of the failure of biomedicine to address the primary health care needs of poor and minority communities. He located the "need" for primary health care in general, and CHAs in particular, in the economic conditions and other forces that kept families in Brighton Square marginalized. Weaver argued that conventional health care is ill-equipped to deal with the wide-ranging needs of those who inhabit the margins of society. He saw the figure of the CHA as a necessary proxy for the doctor in determining "need" and linking families with services. Weaver described to me the social determinants of health he observed and the limitations individual physicians face in affecting individuals' behavior:

> So we, people who work in communities that are outside the mainstream, understand very well that our folks don't do as well, regardless of the measure, . . . they don't do as well. So we know that . . . living in a community where most of the people are poor is not healthy. Living in a community where most of the people don't finish high school is not healthy. There's really good evidence. We live in a community where there are probably more people connected to the prison system than there are connected to colleges. We live in a community where the police are looked at as antagonists. All of these things are directly related to health outcomes. So, if I spent all my time just sitting in an exam room with an individual, who has many things going on in her life, . . . they have children in trouble or household violence or . . . , you know, when those things are going on, whether you're on a twelve-hundred-calorie diet or an eighteen-hundred-calorie diet, or whether you even take your insulin . . . , they just fall in importance.

What is needed, Weaver suggested, is an outreach program that relies on *members* of these "communities that are outside the mainstream" to provide information about available health resources to every family in the hopes that they will take advantage of them. This lay health outreach worker model relies on the social relationships among individuals to try to mobilize the sick to seek better care, at the same time that it relies on the poor and sick themselves to actually avail themselves of those resources. CHAs, as "members" of these communities, are best situated to both diagnose needs and perform linkages between family members, agencies, churches, and the health care provider. Interestingly, Weaver calls this approach a "different method of [illness] management," in which what is provided is not care *per se* but *information*:

> Our goal is to minimize the difference. . . . So therefore, although it's important for the person who's ill to have medical care, . . . we also have to know where [that] fits in the big scheme. So we have to work on other methods to improve the health of the community. Those things are not well understood in this country. We feel that the way to do it is to move on from the most sick people [to] a different method of management. In other words, it's not the doctor and the patient in the exam room, it's the patient, the person with the illness, and their nurse case manager who has them in mind, in the setting that they're in, which is their home, their church, or their elder center, or their something, and over a long period of time, providing the information that that person needs to do well with their chronic illness. That's how you do it.

The larger CHA program was modeled on this approach of population-based health care and outreach, but each agency made modifications according to its political orientation and funding arrangements. Thus the Brighton Square approach was only one among several implementations of the CHA program but was the most successful one in winning funding for their program. They were able to support six CHAs with full-time, competitive salaries and full benefits, and thus elected not to submit proposals with TCHC and Helping the Black Family for WtW funding, as outlined in the following chapter.[20] TCHC and Helping the Black Family took a more empowerment-based approach that placed greater emphasis on the personal and professional development of individual health advocates and was based less strictly on mapping zones. Both agencies were able to pay their CHAs through their agreements with the WtW program, paying them six dollars to seven dollars per hour. In fact, one rationale for the WtW funding application was the argument that the program's initial funding from the Robert Wood Johnson Foundation could pay a program coordinator at each partner agency but not CHAs, or CHAs but not a coordinator.

This chapter shows how NGOs, states, and other bodies have produced "communities" as a unit of intervention. I suggest that the CHAs are shaped as idealized citizens—community organizers—in part by means

---

20. The Brighton Square Community Health Coalition, and thus the Brighton Square CHAs, were supported by Fielding Hospital and therefore were written into a wider array of both research and service proposals. The convergence of research and service as a means of governing communities is addressed further in Part II.

of the discursive opposition between agency and community. I describe the various meanings of the term *community* and look at its co-inflection with language and ethnic identity to explore by what discursive means the citizenship of CHAs is enabled. The following chapter presents the modifications made to the CHA program under WtW funding and introduces a different kind of ideal: the productive citizen.

3

Neoliberalism at Work

Contemporary Scenarios of Governmental
Reforms in Public Health and Social Work

Seven months into my fieldwork in 1998, the CHA program began to receive federal welfare reform monies for operating support. As the health center began to take part in the nationwide reallocation of resources aimed at moving welfare recipients into the "world of work," this new phase brought many changes to the CHA program, which had been in operation less than a year before it received this new grant. The Access Enterprise, as the county's Welfare-to-Work (WtW) project was called, made CHA coordinators subject to new regimes of accountability. Funding requirements specified many features of the CHA program that had previously been left up to the agencies' discretion, including the target population, what constituted "training," program duration, and other key features. WtW instituted new relationships with other agencies and changes in hierarchies of relationship among agencies. As each CHA program coordinator tried to position their CHAs to receive the maximum possible benefits from WtW (and there were some, if not many), they were accountable to a new model of "helping" based more in the logic of verification and enforcement (Cruikshank 1999; Bane and Ellwood 1994) than in community empowerment. While earlier welfare policies allowed more flexibility and discretion for case managers to determine their clients' needs and issue resources, the logic of verification required caseworkers to generate paper trails in order to be able to defend their decisions in the face of the always-eventual audit (Power 1994; Carlen 2008). Finally, and most significantly, a new population, the so-called hardest-to-serve, was constituted and specified as appropriate (indeed, the only) candidates to be CHAs. New mechanisms of accounting tracked the progress of these "hardest to serve" welfare recipients through the CHA training and program, ideally culminating in their placement into full-time permanent employment.

The WtW grant funded most of the original partners on the CHA project (TCHC, Helping the Black Family, and El Pueblo, all under the umbrella of Healthy Communities, Inc. [HCI]), but also introduced new "collaborators" in the citywide initiative. In 1998, the city of Thornton disbursed approximately $2.4 million in federal welfare reform funds to local agencies through a request for proposals. WtW in Alistair County was governed through a complex series of contracts and subcontracts flowing from the state through ever-smaller, more privatized units. WtW essentially amounted to an elaborate job training program, albeit one in which clients are "empowered" in part through the language of consumerism. Calling clients *consumers*, for example, supposedly returns the power of choice to those traditionally constructed as dependent on the state. Correspondingly, the *point of sale* is the company or organization that employs the welfare recipient. The Job Training Unit, a county agency already well funded to provide a range of job training programs, was the main contractor for the WtW program.[1] The Job Training Unit then subcontracted with HCI, the umbrella agency for the CHA program. HCI's partner agencies and sub-subcontractors—TCHC, Helping the Black Family, and the Brighton Square Community Health Coalition—were responsible for the day-to-day management of women on welfare. Staff members of these agencies felt that a qualitative change had taken place with the advent of WtW funding in the nature and meaning of their work.

This chapter sketches the broad outlines of changes in government that help explain why an empowerment-based program such as the CHA program would apply for and receive WtW funds. After first tracing the contours of the new populations (the so-called hardest-to-serve and those merely "at risk" of welfare dependency) constructed by WtW, I explore a set of concepts that served as focal points for two different approaches to governing the poor. The concepts of *empowerment, self-sufficiency,* and *participation* were mobilized by both the WtW approach and the earlier community health approach to the CHA program, with at times divergent meanings and powerful consequences. In the analysis that follows,

---

1. In Massachusetts, WtW created a new bureaucracy *parallel* to the state's own welfare offices. As part of politicians' promises to "end welfare as we know it," WtW was not administered through states' existing public aid offices but rather through private industry councils (PICs), which distributed WtW funds through contracts and subcontracts with vendors such as HCI. Additional WtW case managers were funded at PICs as a supplement to existing caseworkers employed by the state welfare office.

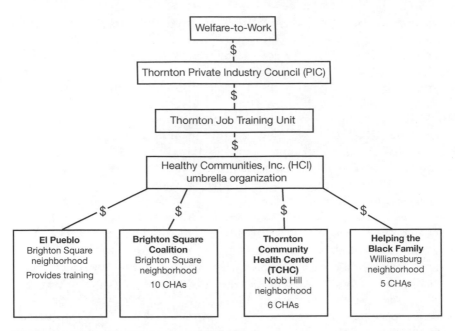

Welfare-to-Work funding for the CHA program.

I compare the *empowerment model* with the notion of *personal responsibility* that suffuses welfare reform. Both empowerment and personal responsibility hinge on the active *participation* of women on welfare, invoking a relationship of governing between the health advocate, the community members, and the welfare agency. As empowered community organizers who were meant to transfer that process of empowerment to bureaucratically and ethnically constituted communities, CHAs were interpellated into ambiguous processes of social and political representation. I examine these concepts as nodes of language and practice that reveal the relationships of governance active in both phases of the CHA program.

What Problems Did Welfare-to-Work Solve?

How did an empowerment-based, public health outreach program become a job training program for women on welfare? To answer this question, we can consider the problems facing the CHA program, to which WtW would appear to be a solution. WtW funding solved problems plaguing Thornton Community Health Center's relationship with the local welfare department. For participants to receive perks such as child care assistance and bus vouchers from the welfare office, the CHA program had to qualify first as "community service" and later, under WtW, as a job training program, defined as any "work experience program" for welfare recipients that led to guaranteed job placement. WtW came with an agreement from the state welfare department that all WtW programs constituted job training insofar as the program itself guaranteed a job, albeit a time-limited one, for every participant. However, the fix was only temporary; after just six months of WtW funding, the clinic had to assume 100 percent responsibility for CHA salaries, following a payment schedule in which WtW paid a decreasing proportion of salary costs.[2]

Specifying Populations

While it solved certain problems, the decision to pursue WtW funding led to new ones. Stringent criteria defined who was eligible to participate in WtW. One loudly trumpeted innovation in the federal legislation was its focus on the so-called hardest-to-serve welfare recipients. Public debates around welfare reform in 1996 focused on welfare recipients who remain on welfare and who are seen as resistant to education and training, despite the repeated mobilization of statistics by advocates that the average length of stay for a welfare recipient is two years.[3]

---

2. None of the agencies in the CHA collaboration had adequate funding to guarantee permanent jobs for the CHAs. In a report to HCI, the umbrella funding recipient of RWJF funds (see note 2 in Chapter 2), TCHC staff wrote, "The project has suffered from its timing insofar as it coincided with welfare reform, which negatively affected it at the outset since the original conditions under which the RWJ CHA grant was written changed. While original expectations were that the CHAs would be made up in part of welfare recipients obligated to perform twenty hours a week of community service, welfare reform has changed who is eligible or obligated to do community service. This change has affected our pool of applicants and led to the requirement that we provide paid positions for our CHAs before we were able to. We coped with these difficulties by overextending ourselves and putting the CHAs on payroll before a solid source of funding was identified." HCI's report to the foundation included this item in response to a question regarding "internal problems encountered during the year": "The project design counted on the use of people in transition from welfare to work as the principal audience from which to recruit CHAs. There was a significant shift in the administration of these transitional programs away from activities that support 'community service' to 'work first.' [For more on "work first," see the discussion later in this chapter.] With this shift the 'soft' training program, as we were viewed, was not sufficient under this new policy. As a result, we have begun an adaptation of the recruitment, training, and delivery program." TCHC ended its participation in the CHA program in 2001.

3. Furthermore, most welfare recipients are *not* long-term recipients. A fact sheet available in Thornton's welfare office, however, explained that long-term recipients (two years or more) aggregate in the caseload over time so that at any given moment most recipients will have received welfare for more than two years. The Welfare Information Network (WIN), a nonprofit research organization, suggested that universal work requirements for people on welfare could "'smoke out' those with special needs simply by subjecting all recipients to some form of work related activity" (Kramer 1998, 6). This move uses the marketplace to sort recipients' capabilities and locates the "barriers to employment" in the individuals rather than the market.

The "hardest to serve," as defined by legislators, are long-term welfare recipients (receiving benefits for more than two years) who have at least two of the following three characteristics:

1. Lacking high school diploma or GED[4]
2. In need of substance abuse treatment
3. Poor work history (no more than three consecutive months' employment during the previous year)

WtW legislation further mandated that 70 percent of federal funds must be spent "serving" these individuals. Of these three criteria, the most important in practice was the lack of a high school degree. TCHC employed no welfare recipients who acknowledged having a substance abuse problem. Therefore, if the CHAs already on staff were to be supported by the WtW grant, they had to lack a high school diploma. Unfortunately, all of the CHAs working for the clinic except one had completed high school or gotten a GED. While the clinic was able to keep two of these CHAs using its "own" funds, several CHAs were fired because they did not meet these criteria and because other funding was inadequate to support their salaries.

The implementation of WtW at TCHC was marked by chaos as CHAs worried about their futures with the agency and the health center tried to hire new, replacement, "hardest to serve" welfare recipients as CHAs. This upheaval affected the structure of feeling of the WtW program at TCHC, as CHA administrators justified their actions by appealing to sources of power higher than themselves, and participants felt subject to a bureaucracy that operated according to whim, not by any logic they could understand. How could program staff explain giving jobs to welfare recipients, training them to be community change agents, then letting them go because they had *too much* education? CHAs responded by lashing out at all aspects of the program. Viviana, an outspoken CHA, complained to me, "When we came here, we had no housing [no office space of their own], we had no structure and . . . we have no leadership. Everything and everyone is out of control. We do what we can when we can, whenever, but it's not like, set." Viviana put her finger on a key aspect of a program plagued by disorganization. As Viviana pointed out, when the health advocates completed their training at the local community college, they worked out of a series of temporary offices because TCHC did not have a space ready for them. This bumpy beginning was followed almost immediately by layoffs of CHAs who did not meet the WtW "hardest to serve" criteria.

---

4. The GED (general equivalency degree) is a national substitute for a high school diploma obtained by passing an exam. People who drop out of high school usually can take a class in order to obtain their GED.

Looking back on his decision to pursue WtW funding, TCHC executive director George Williams commented in an interview with me:

> One of the reasons that I was so adamant that we . . . join them in terms of the proposal for the Welfare-to-Work project, so that we could get support for these individuals going on to do other things, was that I believe you don't do people good when you bring them in, have them do some work, and then you let them go. So how do they experience us? If we're a community health center that our mandate is to provide services, mind, body, and spirit, then we are exploiting people if we do that. . . . There has to be consistency between what we do and what we say. So if we say that community health centers provide services that allow people their dignity and their self-worth, et cetera, et cetera, then I think the people we employ, we have to do the same thing. We have to go the extra mile for people. So now we're employing people who don't have skills, so we have to go the extra mile in terms of bringing them in and providing opportunities and support for them.

Williams seemed to believe that WtW would have provided additional support for CHAs. Perhaps he was not aware of the population specifications that would prevent most of the CHAs on staff at the time from remaining with the program. Whatever the case, the consequences of the decision to take part in the WtW program were completely different from what Williams anticipated here.

The confusion introduced by WtW funding was in stark contrast to the implementation process described in the WtW policy and procedures manual handed out in the first meeting for new case managers. In fact, Nikki Sparrow and Imani Riyad, the CHA program coordinators, objected to the rigor and specificity of the new program because they were accustomed to the latitude implied by utter confusion. For the health advocates, on the other hand, the advent of the WtW program only confirmed their suspicions that TCHC staff were in league with the welfare office because of the greater degree of collaboration required between the CHA program coordinators and welfare caseworkers. Accustomed to rampant disorganization and incomprehensible bureaucracy from the welfare system, the health advocates were disgusted but not surprised by the health center's inability to provide a workspace, timely paychecks, and other features of regular employment. Each partner agency had similar experiences of large or small crises around payment, space, eligibility, and so on. The WtW program introduced new procedures with their own contradictions, complexities, and confusions that program managers sought to navigate as they worked to turn newly minted community organizers into productive citizens.

Creating Productive Citizens through Welfare-to-Work

The Personal Responsibility and Work Opportunity Reconciliation Act of 1996 enacts many features of neoliberal social policy, including a reliance on marketplace logic, the valorization of self-sufficiency and the creation of productive citizens in place of previous governmental concern with social welfare, the emergence of new forms and territories of government, and the implementation of new networks of power such as public-private partnerships. Enrolling in the WtW program meant agencies and individuals became entangled in new regimes of power that operated on the CHA program's existing language of ethnicity, community, and health in novel, sometimes uncomfortable ways. These changes have had a deep impact on social work and public health programs such as the CHA program.

Neoliberal policies have transformed the notion of guaranteed economic welfare as a political or social right associated with the liberal welfare state into something more akin to a wage, a benefit that must be earned in order for the citizen to perform as a consumer in the neoliberal order (Rose 1999). Work requirements first appeared in the United States in the early 1980s, though work requirements have long been attached to various forms of public assistance elsewhere (see, e.g., Poovey 1995). In 1994, Massachusetts's welfare reform law also included work requirements but mapped out broader categories of exemption than later federal requirements. The Personal Responsibility and Work Opportunity Reconciliation Act of 1996 (PRWORA) enacted the most sweeping reforms to welfare assistance seen in thirty years, ending the federal entitlement program AFDC (Aid to Families with Dependent Children) and rerouting the funds to a series of block grants to the states. WtW required all welfare recipients to be engaged in paid work and dramatically restricted the categories of recipients who could be entirely exempt from work (Brodkin 1997, 25).

Rather than reorganizing state welfare offices, WtW was implemented instead through public-private partnerships and other new networks. Public-private partnerships allow states to disclaim governing authority while participating in problem-solving efforts governed by the language and logic of the market. As governments demur to directly provide services, authority circulates through networks, contested and renegotiated according to flows of resources.[5] The various state and nonstate actors in these partnerships are tied together through networks of contracts and subcontracts. Sanford Schram (2000) discusses "contractual discourse" as

---

5. These partnerships constitute a new form of governance in which the state itself is now "simply one element . . . in multiple circuits of power, connecting a diversity of authorities and forces, within a whole variety of complex assemblages" (Rose 1999, 5). In the partnership governing Thornton's WtW program, TCHC and other agencies receiving WtW funds are known as "vendors" because they provide job training services not to welfare recipients but to the state's welfare bureaucracy.

a productive discourse in which political subjects are rearticulated as consumers in a post-welfare state that functions more like a marketplace than a state. In fact, the notion of contract has permeated the very provision of welfare benefits itself. It is increasingly common that individuals must sign a contract with a welfare agency stipulating the "rights and responsibilities" of "both parties" in order to receive benefits. Contracts such as these are an enduring disciplinary technique of welfare reform (Gilbert 2002; Schram 2000). Welfare recipients' responsibilities may range far beyond the economic to school, child raising, or other family matters, revealing how welfare reform penetrates many aspects of recipients' lives in the name of more and better *self*-government.[6] As a political relationship, however, the contractual relationship between consumer and health care provider, for example, is fundamentally economic because there is no institutional or legal position for the consumer except that which can be defended in civil court.

These forms of a restructured welfare state are built on a new equation between the best interests of society and the best interests of the market. Market rationalities make their appearance in new areas of government that were previously defined and understood through notions of the social good or welfare. A hallmark of this economic-capitalist framework is the use of the keyword *choice* throughout social and health care services (Rose 1999, 141–142). The discourse of welfare reform seeks to reattribute agency to welfare recipients, typically described as dependent and inactive, through the language of choice. People receiving welfare benefits are now offered "choices," even when they appear in the form of work requirements and the options are preselected and limited. James Riccio and Yeheskel Hasenfeld suggest that "giving recipients a choice of participation treats them as 'consumers' rather than 'objects' to be processed. This puts an onus on welfare department staff to 'market' their services to recipients, which, as in the private economy, can lead to higher quality services" (1996, 518). As well, community participation is sometimes described in terms that reposition or refigure the patient or client as a "consumer."[7] The language of consumerism denies the position of *client*

---

6. For example, a "personal responsibility contract" might include "commitments and agreements ranging from parenting, to family budget management, to job search and workplace goals. Typically, . . . the applicant is required to make 10 job contacts and document them before being eligible to attend the orientation meeting" for eligible welfare recipients (Nathan and Gais 1999, 24).

7. Anne Lovell and Sandra Cohn extend this analysis to a study of rehabilitation programs for the mentally ill. They highlight the rhetoric of "choice" featured in a New York program for mentally ill homeless people to show how it serves as a means by which consuming subjects are created from these most unlikely consumers. "The image of 'choices unlimited' erases the unequal footing created by economic and cultural capital, while conjuring up the enterprising individual" (1998, 12).

and introduces new notions of accountability into the provider-patient relationship.[8]

Various authors (Osborne 1997; Porter 1995; Willging 2005) have tracked the appearance of these and other keywords previously seen only in domains of management and business, such as *accountability, performance standards, outcomes, deliverables, rewards linked to performance, contracts and competition,* and *budget discipline.* These terms signal the application of frameworks and techniques from management to new realms concerned with the government of subjects, the provision of care, and other diverse areas. Under both funding regimes (RWJF and WtW) for the CHA program, new accounting and data collection requirements focused on documenting program outcomes in order to receive funding. CHAs who completed the empowerment-based training programs described earlier found themselves, once at work, faced with service delivery reports and many other accountability requirements. HCI, the umbrella agency for the CHA program, led an effort to institute outcome funding, in which money is paid only on completion of "deliverables" or outcomes. Imani Riyad, the CHA coordinator for Helping the Black Family, another site of the program, wondered how she would pay for her staff who were supposed to deliver these outcomes when the money would be paid from HCI to each of its three subcontractors only on completion. Helping the Black Family was paid only after they placed 70 percent of their CHAs in permanent, full-time employment. Niara Kadar, the CHA trainer who worked closely with all three agencies participating in the CHA program, forecast that agencies would have to pick up the slack by providing services and follow-up to clients who may have had more support before welfare reform. Kadar explained:

> Now what we did when we were working with that kind of a grant [that was funded through outcomes] was we were able to fulfill the grant before the end of the year, which meant you worked very,

---

8. For example, an article in *Public Administration Review* (Rago 1996) describes the restructuring of the Texas Department of Mental Health when it rewrote its mission statement to resemble a more participatory model. Using the language of *consumer* rather than *client*, they chose as their guide the Total Quality Management model, a popular management approach in the early 1990s, driven by the ideals of "consumer choice" and "customer satisfaction." Since reformers in the department wanted to "orient the service system toward the consumer," Texas mental health agencies first needed to make their patients into consumers. These changes are clearly market driven and reflect the need to "quickly respond to the choices made" by their "consumers." Their mission statement also calls for *actively participating* consumers "in shaping the services available in the community" (Rago 1996, 228). In addition, some health care advocates have argued that as "consumers" rather than patients, people would have more bargaining power in relation to health care providers (Reeder 1978). However, the language of *caveat emptor* also implies a loss of governmental regulation or protections for the buyer.

very, very hard, and I'm sure that they do. An outcome for them is thirty days on the job for the person, which means whatever happened on the thirty-first day, who cares? You made your thirty days; that's all we care about. We keep checking with you until you hit thirty; when you hit thirty-four and everything falls apart, you're on your own. They made their money and they're happy; they had a success, and they're on to the next. But with the folks that they're talking about in these high-risk groups that they're bringing in [for Welfare-to-Work], the follow-up has to be a year. But there's no money or mechanisms built in for them to follow those women for a year and continue giving them support or have a case manager or somebody that's out there working for them. So they probably need to rely pretty heavily on these community-based agencies that are going to be able to do the follow-up.

Reframing the delivery of services in terms of "products" or "deliverables" does have human costs, Kadar emphasized, and only displaces the burden of those costs onto other NGOs. By requiring only that individuals remain "attached" to the job market for at least one year (to be counted as an "outcome") instead of maintaining the *same job* for a year, welfare reform fostered the flexibility for both workers and employers that is paramount in a quickly changing market. Individual employers were therefore not required to be responsible for a welfare recipient for an entire year but could transfer that responsibility with no consequences. Linking the development of government and the population with that of the market means that hierarchy and fixed roles must give way to flexibility and multitasking ability (Walters 1997). Accordingly, workers must be ready to avail themselves of many possible work roles on short notice. There was little emphasis on specific or long-term job training in WtW but instead a proliferation of programs aimed at creating willing, malleable, and agreeable workers. For example, "job readiness" trainings that I observed substituted what Sanford Schram (2000) calls the "soft skills" of customer service (how to dress, how to arrive on time, how to handle authority) for actual job training, reflecting changes in the burgeoning postindustrial service economy.[9]

---

9. In a historical discussion that could easily apply to contemporary views of welfare recipients, Giovanna Procacci (1991) argues that public disgust for "paupers" or the poor in nineteenth-century England was based not so much on their *dependence* on the largesse of society but on their *independence*—their unwillingness to avail themselves of work opportunities in the marketplace: "The economic critique which reproaches public assistance for maintaining islands of dependence in a society organized around the 'free' disposal of one's self, is actually an attack on those existing social ties that are seen as obsolete . . . precisely because of the specific way in which they mediate dependence: forming people into a bloc, resisting the 'free' circulation of individuals in the network of the labour market" (1991, 161).

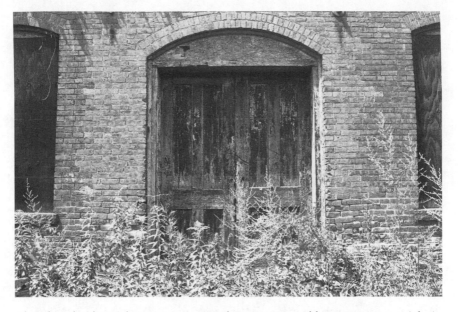

Abandoned industrial sites, some more than a century old, are a common sight in Thornton. *(Photograph courtesy of Amanda Quinby.)*

Rather than liberation from bureaucratic red tape, privatization of welfare added a new layer of bureaucracy to an already complex process for receiving benefits. WtW case managers had to move between two duplicative yet separate bureaucracies in addition to their "home" agency or company: the welfare office, and WtW. Even the apparently simple act of getting a participant enrolled in a WtW program required herculean efforts by the WtW case manager, who shepherded a potential participant through a maze of screenings, assessments, and intake procedures by which eligibility in newly defined populations was ascertained. The WtW case manager had to martial resources from the Thornton Private Industry Council as well as the welfare office while maintaining constant contact with the participant to ensure that she was not lost during the entire tortuous process.

Welfare-to-Work: New Regimes of Labor, Structures of Accountability, and the Formation of Ethical Subjects

So you're throwing into a pot that's already bubbling around, not really knowing what the heck you're cooking, a whole new set of ingredients. I just don't know. —Niara Kadar

The political rationalities associated with neoliberalism are framed in moral terms as well as economic ones—or rather, economic rationalities themselves operate with a moral force (Rose 1999, 27). The condition of self-sufficiency takes on moral as well as economic value, while dependency on government benefits maintains its long-term stigmatization. The truth of neoliberalism can be summed up in two mantras: the market is always right, and small government is better. Welfare reform proponents describe neoliberal policy developments as making society *more* democratic rather than less by virtue of their inclusivity, arguing that people who receive welfare do not want to do so; they would prefer to work and cannot feel like equal citizens until they do work.[10] Legislators who argue that work requirements simply help welfare recipients achieve what "we" know "they" want attribute agency to welfare recipients in interesting ways. In numerous domains since neoliberal reforms began in the 1980s, policy changes seeking to remove the state as gatekeeper cite evidence that barriers have been removed, discrimination is illegal, and we are all, ipso facto, equal on the terrain of the market.

The governmental logic of welfare reform in the United States moved from the categorization of recipients by type of need or disability to the linking of benefits to the overarching goal of productive activity. The ultimate goal of WtW was, of course, paid employment, and most program practices were aimed at positioning recipients for low-level service jobs. An individual who is not actually working participates in structured job searches.[11] An individual who is in a WtW program is allowed to maintain certain benefits while working, and a case manager enforces his or her adherence to attendance and other requirements. Welfare recipients are encouraged toward this goal of self-management with the assistance of their caseworkers. Welfare or unemployment case managers supervise the formation of a self-disciplining and motivated subject as a citizen of the active society (Walters 1997; Dean 1997).[12]

Treating the Risk of Dependency through Work

After using 70 percent of WtW funding for the "hardest to serve," the remainder of federal funds could be spent on welfare recipients who merely have any three of the *"characteristics* of welfare dependency."

---

10. Nikolas Rose characterizes this view thus: "Not only does [welfare] represent a drain on individual incomes and on national finances; it also stifles responsibility, inhibits risk taking, [and] induces dependency. Hence it actually *exacerbates*, rather than reducing the division between the included and the excluded" (1999, 159; emphasis added). See also Hyatt 2001 for further analysis of neoliberal views of the welfare state.

11. Stephanie Limoncelli (2002) gives an excellent description of one such program in California.

12. "Through these practices, the individual *no longer claims a benefit* but becomes a client of various agencies, seeking and obeying the directions of pastoral agents, and receiving an allowance *conditional on establishing a particular relation to the self*" (Dean 1997, 575–576).

Interestingly, while the features of "hardest to serve" were set by federal legislators, the specification of this second category was left up to the states to determine. In Massachusetts, there were fourteen "characteristics of welfare dependency":

1. high school dropout
2. low reading and/or math skills
3. substance abuse
4. lacks/poor work history
5. limited English proficiency
6. homeless
7. more than one dependent
8. disabled
9. disabled family member
10. offender
11. public/subsidized housing
12. pregnant/parenting youth
13. non-English high school diploma
14. Enterprise Community zone/high poverty census tract[13]

This list is sufficiently broad to cover most poor people in Thornton, and many nonpoor people as well. By creating an apparently free-associated list of characteristics of poor people, *all* remaining welfare recipients who do not fit in the "hardest to serve" category can be described as "having the characteristics of welfare dependency." Thus simply being on welfare, if not simply being poor, is tantamount to being at risk for "welfare dependency."[14] In this policy move specifying another new population, "dependency" expands to cover all welfare recipients and many poor people as well. The notion of dependency was constantly referenced in public debate as justification for welfare reform in the mid-1990s, to the extent that its meaning became overladen with gendered and racialized ideological associations.[15] Dependency is the rhetorical opposite of the notion of the *self-sufficient* citizen-subject that animates federal welfare reform (Schram 2000). Social work scholar Sanford Schram argues that the 1996 welfare

13. The list is from a handout titled "Request for Proposals: Welfare-to-Work" distributed at a meeting of the Thornton Job Training Institute and prospective applicants for WtW funding, January 23, 1998.
14. In a wide-ranging review, Deborah Lupton (1999) draws together the work of several major theorists on risk to show how risk has become an instrument for the government of populations. Here, the designation of an entire population of poor people as "at risk" for the stigmatized condition of dependency enables new modes of intervention in the lives of the poor who seek income assistance, including "work first" and other requirements described further later in this chapter.
15. Nancy Naples (1997) analyzes the deployment of dependency discourse in the 1987–1988 congressional welfare reform debates; see also Fraser and Gordon 1994.

reform law medicalizes dependency to an unprecedented degree, making the receipt of welfare benefits a result of personal flaws or deficiencies that must be treated through techniques of government such as work placement, self-esteem therapy, drug treatment, and other kinds of programs, "creat[ing] the conditions for moving welfare from an income redistribution scheme to a behavior modification regime" (Schram 2000, 60).[16]

Further, encoded within items such as "more than one dependent" or living in a "high poverty census tract" or "public housing" is the imagined, stereotypical welfare queen. Diane Thomas, a CHA, felt that this stereotype was the lens through which she was being seen as she walked down the street in her predominantly white, working-class neighborhood:

> They had a concert in the park down there, and, you know, I didn't realize there are so many white people in [this town]. [*Laughs.*] There's a lot of them. So I'm walking up Main Street to go to the store, and I'm just seeing all these people staring at me. Automatically, they assume, black female, welfare recipient, fifty million children. And this is how I'm thinking they looking at me. 'Cause I had Lisa's son with me when I went. And that's the idea they have of black people in general. But, just as I said, yes, at this point I still am on AFDC, but I work just as well as the next person.

Thomas felt that the stereotype of "black female, welfare recipient" adhered to her and she was compelled to assert her ability to *work* in response to the stereotype. If stereotypes about women on welfare are effects of accounting practices such as those that define "hardest to serve," they have even broader sequelae than what Thomas describes here. The typical liberal response to such stereotypes denies them as unfair and unreal. Governmentality theorists such as Barbara Cruikshank (1999) show how stereotypes like this do not emerge from generalizations from the actual bodies of actual women on welfare, but instead come into being as a result of the accounting and audit practices mobilized by the state's concern for verification.

Lists such as the preceding one specifying the population "at risk" for welfare dependency are exactly the kind of accounting practices Cruikshank describes. Rather than simply debunking stereotypes about crafty welfare queens with stories of the virtuous poor, Cruikshank urges us to look instead at how the welfare queen came to be, the way in which she came to have a body or an image that we picture when we hear her name. To this

---

16. However, "the problem" of poverty has been located in faulty individuals throughout various historical periods, with corresponding solutions that involve different kinds of modifications of the poor. See Lubove 1965, Poovey 1995, and Gwendolyn Mink in Gordon 1990, among others.

end, then, we should examine the effects of programs such as WtW on the women who take part in them. It is through these kinds of governmental practices that stereotypes can be said to become embodied as they act on the bodies of women who are subject to them, supporting the pernicious imaginary of "the welfare queen" that drives contemporary welfare policy.

Finding the Hardest to Serve

Finding welfare recipients categorized as "hardest to serve" was a difficult task in and of itself. Miriam Butler, WtW coordinator for the city of Thornton, was a petite African American woman who granted me an interview in her rented office next door to a coffee shop. Shaking her head in dismay, she acknowledged that the few characteristics qualifying someone as "hardest to serve" would limit the number of people agencies would be able to enroll into WtW. An additional challenge in working with this population was its refusal to constitute itself as a population, insofar as drug users may reject the self-representation that is called for in that process.[17] Butler explained:

> The intent is to serve those people who are the hardest to serve. Those are people, the drug addicts that have been on welfare all of their life, [who] have no work skills, and I qualify that because I hate it when people say somebody has no skills because that's just not true. But they have no work experience, none whatsoever, and they've got millions of barriers, maybe four or five children; it's just—these are the people that the welfare offices have not—no one has ever tried to deal with. They really wanted to focus the money on those people. . . . Those are the people that are probably on and off welfare, have some skills, just need a little push, a little help. . . . [So] it's making it really difficult to serve anybody. People are not going to come forward and admit to substance abuse. . . . So it's hard to find these hardest-to-serve people. And when you find them, realistically, they're not going to be in a position where you can serve them, because they're going to need treatment, you know; they need counseling, they need [drug] treatment, they need all of that first before they're even ready to think about looking for a job. So yeah, it makes it very tough. Very tough.

While the adult education model used by CHA trainers held that *every person* had relevant life experience valuable to her role as outreach worker,

---

17. Part II presents examples of drug user organizing around harm reduction, however, where at-risk populations are articulated in response to health threats such as HIV and hepatitis.

welfare staff, in contrast, viewed the "hardest to serve" requirements as equivalent to "scraping the bottom of the barrel," as another welfare administrator memorably put it. At the same time, everyone recognized the difficulty of recruiting the group of people thus defined and motivating them to participate in job training programs.

Enrolling new CHAs into the WtW program helped initiate individual welfare recipients into a new population of "hardest to serve." But the enrollment process was so complex and arcane, it seemed designed to *discourage* participation by the very people (disorganized, no work history) it supposedly sought to enroll. For example, Carleen Morris, twenty years old with an eighteen-month-old daughter, was already on staff as a CHA when the WtW program began at TCHC. For the cost of her salary to be picked up by the WtW grant, and for the program to continue supporting her as a CHA, Carleen had to be enrolled as the single "30 percent person" allowed in this program of six welfare recipients, since she already had a GED. First, TCHC had to ask her welfare worker to recommend her to the "administrative oversight" agency, the Thornton Private Industry Council (PIC). The PIC then sent Carleen a letter informing her of her appointment for "intake testing," including reading and math evaluations. Knowing the intake criteria, the CHA coordinator advised her to not score too high on these tests. Carleen said that she never got the letter, and she learned of the appointment by calling the PIC to confirm her eligibility. She showed up at the PIC on the designated day, only to learn that she was supposed to be at the welfare office, not the PIC office, for this evaluation. She found a ride over to the welfare office but arrived fifteen minutes late for the appointment, only to be told that late arrivals were not admitted. She went home, frustrated. Nikki Sparrow, the CHA program coordinator at TCHC, called to reschedule her appointment and bullied the PIC administrator into coming to the health center for the evaluation rather than sending Carleen to the welfare office again. The test at last completed, Carleen then had to complete an entirely new round of personnel paperwork because though she was employed at the same agency, she was now being paid by another agency. Unlike many new CHAs recruited from the "hardest to serve" category, Carleen was highly motivated to keep the job that she had held for the past five months. However, she could easily have been lost in the confusing series of letters and missed appointments her enrollment into WtW entailed.

A handout distributed at an orientation meeting for new WtW coordinators represents the WtW program as a complex loop designed to move participants through an "employment ladder" eventually leading to stable employment at a living-wage job. The boxes on the left show the administrative steps required to move a participant through the system.[18] The ovals

18. Note that in this "bird's-eye view" diagram the last step, "Postplacement," does not actually lead to independence but back to eligibility/assessment. Despite the best intentions

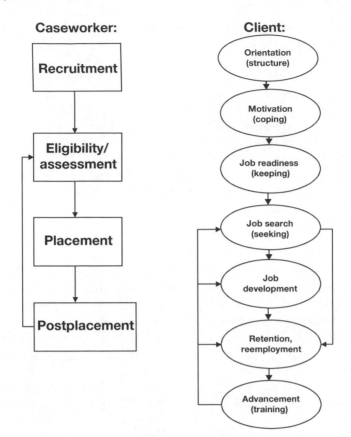

Caseworker:

Recruitment

Eligibility/ assessment

Placement

Postplacement

Client:

Orientation (structure)

Motivation (coping)

Job readiness (keeping)

Job search (seeking)

Job development

Retention, reemployment

Advancement (training)

Bird's-eye view of the Welfare-to-Work customer flow.

on the right show the process from the participant's perspective, describing the responsibilities of the participant (with the case manager's assistance) along the way. A new, active attitude toward employment can be seen in the verbs "coping," "keeping," and "seeking." Even simply not getting fired from or quitting a job is a step—"retention." It is worth noting that training and "advancement," while always mentioned in the WtW literature, are the last step, almost an afterthought, in this process.

"Work First"

Once found and enrolled, people on welfare who signed up for WtW were placed directly into jobs without first receiving any training or education,

---

to "end welfare as we know it," this seems to indicate an understanding that clients will always be clients, always eligible for reassessment.

because WtW is a "work first" program. According to the Thornton PIC's call for proposals, "The best way for a person to learn about work is to work." Once employed, a WtW participant was eligible for services such as basic education, skills training, English as a second language classes, and so on. Attending college, or even getting a GED, is no longer an "approved activity." But training *before* work was understood as and restricted to so-called job readiness activities, such as classroom instruction on showing up for work on time, appropriate attire, and arranging for child care. These job readiness programs were oriented to the level of the mundane, practical "skills and attitudes" that welfare recipients were thought to lack.

Job training components were retermed "Work Experience," for those who had none, and "Supported Work," for those who had some work experience but still needed to maintain benefits while working. In a planning meeting for WtW case managers, Kadar addressed this issue bluntly: "So, the people we're supposed to [hire] are the hardest to employ, the ones who have never worked, and the first thing they're supposed to do is work?" Ironic smiles around the table recognized her point. Sanford Schram (2000) and others (e.g., Korteweg 2003) note that PRWORA was built on the assumption that the mere act of working itself functions therapeutically for welfare recipients, who are presumably (and, in the definitions of the populations described earlier, categorically) without skills or work experience.[19] In an in-depth interview, Imani Riyad, the assistant director at Helping the Black Family, expressed deep cynicism about the "work first" philosophy:

> The notion of working first, to me, is as bizarre as any that I've heard. None of them worked first, the people who thought this up. They all were trained in one way or another through school, through association with folks in their neighborhoods, in their churches, synagogues, wherever they are. Higher education. You know, experiences where they've been able to view other people in the process of doing what they were soon able to do themselves. So, to me, it's an attitude—I don't even know how to name it—it's an elitist, or aloof, attitude that could enable this to even be put into writing. Or ignorance, just total ignorance. And I don't think it's total ignorance 'cause these folks aren't ignorant.

Other administrators I spoke to privately questioned whether it was even possible to locate jobs for welfare recipients completing the WtW pro-

---

19. The "work first" component of WtW was added to the legislation in response to findings that education and training programs were less successful at ending reliance on welfare than programs "stressing immediate labor force attachment" (Nathan and Gais 1999).

gram. Scott Henderson, another WtW coordinator at the PIC, believed that some people were on welfare because they *could not* work, and he questioned the utility of work requirements for these individuals. He noted the irony of an unfunded mandate that required a focus on (rehabilitating) individuals who were substance abusers without any corresponding increase in funding for or access to substance abuse treatment programs.

> Scott: I think that was one of the major assumptions, that there were jobs out there that would pay enough for all of these folks who'd want them. I'm not sure. And I think secondly, sort of an implicit [assumption] is that if these folks really want to work, they can work, and I'm not convinced that everybody on welfare is able to. . . . And I think there are interesting, not inconsistencies, but just contrasts. [For example,] one of the eligibility criteria that might pertain is substance abusers. So on the one hand there's an admission that this is who we need to target, hard-core substance abusers—
> Susan: On the other hand, are there any treatment programs? Right.
> Scott: That was, that's a concern. I think our approach is that we're going to do our best. We're . . . public servants, and we get our paycheck every week because we hopefully provide a public service. And what usually guides our day-to-day activity is whatever law is currently in effect that manipulates society. . . . I'm a realist, though. I have no delusions that we're going to be able to put all these people to work, particularly in sustainable jobs.

"Work first" policies have also been interpreted as an extension of the welfare "contract" that insists on welfare recipient productivity "in exchange for" benefits (Hill and Main 1998), and as an effort to maintain a low-wage workforce for the expanding U.S. service economy (Schram 2000).

From Dependency to Self-Sufficiency: The Self-Fashioning of Welfare Recipients

Once enrolled in the WtW program, new CHAs were given on-the-job training by other CHAs already on staff and eventually training from El Pueblo staff. The El Pueblo training, previously six weeks long and based on participatory education methods, required significant revision to meet WtW mandates. For example, WtW supervisors at the Job Training Unit urged all "vendors" to include a "work readiness" component. The Job Training Unit offered such a component that they called The World of

Work, a two-week pretraining activity designed to socialize participants into practices of self- and time-management (e.g., getting up on time, getting kids to day care, and taking time off). Activities such as these emerge from the belief, common among service providers who work with women on welfare, that welfare recipients lack the personal habits necessary to fit them into the workplace. As Jeanette, a white social worker, told me:

> We're finding out with our population . . . it's hard to change your life habits in a short time. And it's not just that people don't have the skills to get a job; they don't have the know-how to get a job. They don't, they're not in the habit of getting up at seven in the morning, getting the kids ready and out the door, and then being ready to go to work. And see, I was a welfare mother. So I understand this. It was just very difficult to do anything, because most of the time you're saying, "I don't have enough money. I don't have enough help. I don't have a car. I don't have anything. Let me just sit and mull over and have my tea here." And I was lucky it was only tea!

As part of what Nancy Fraser refers to as a "juridical-administrative-therapeutic state apparatus" (1989, 146) the administrative practices of welfare reform work to refashion the habits and practices of the poor to make them more amenable to low-wage work schedules. Another WtW coordinator told me that people on welfare were used to sleeping until they woke up. If, as Sanford Schram argues, the "sickness" of welfare is dependency—inactivity, laziness, the failure to place oneself in the marketplace—then the remedy is work programs and case management practices to "teach" the poor the "skills and behaviors" necessary to articulate one's body into the workplace. These kinds of programs are built on a logic requiring welfare recipients to practice "self-discipline, delayed gratification and modulated pursuit of self-interest" (Schram 2000, 18).

Interventions of this sort often took place through the "pastoral relationship" of the WtW case manager (Dean 1997), who enforced the wide range of behavioral requirements that included living with one's parents if one was a teen parent, keeping one's kids in school, and declaring one's earnings and reporting one's activities properly to the welfare office. CHA program coordinators, serving as WtW caseworkers, generally embraced their responsibility to socialize new health advocates into professional standards of conduct. Despite the special expertise, discussed in Chapter 2, that CHAs held as members of "the community," some agency staff seemed ambivalent toward the presence of traits that marked the health advocates as "community" and sought to mold their behavior to be more professional. For example, Donna, a Caribbean American program

coordinator, complained to me in an interview about the telephone man-
ners of one of her CHAs:

> Susan: What about the impression I got from the training of CHAs
> being community organizers?
> Donna: It is possible, but you know, Susan, with the new Welfare-
> to-Work people, there's a lot of things. I have so much for the
> CHAs, but given the new Welfare-to-Work people, it's going
> to be a difficult task, really . . . because, one particular girl,
> she has a grade level of grade three. And there's a lot of things
> that she doesn't really know in terms of professionalism and
> how to do stuff. It's going to take a lot. And before we can
> actually, say, train them to do CHA work or relay informa-
> tion, we have to teach them the basic things, and it's going to
> take quite a while to do that, you know? Like, for example,
> when she comes, when she speaks on the phone, she speaks
> at the top of her lungs like she's in a marketplace; she knows
> nothing about professionalism. When she's in the office, she
> eats in the front of the office, and she just does things that—
> she doesn't really know. So those are little things that we have
> to be teaching her, and sometimes we have to remind her,
> remind her, remind her. So we're just teaching her office work
> and being professional.

Even their clothing was a contradictory issue: while CHAs were expected
to dress "street" for doing outreach in order to *not* look like a professional and to represent their identity with the community, other clinic staff
objected to the tight blue jeans and tiny baby-doll T-shirts the health advocates wore during agency meetings. Women on welfare who started new,
permanent jobs through WtW received mall coupons to help them get new,
presentable wardrobes. In these and other ways, WtW sought to transform
the subjectivity of welfare recipients who are continuously obliged to work
on themselves.

Empowerment and Personal Responsibility
in the Post-welfare State

In Chapter 2, I showed how the community empowerment model sought
to create CHAs who were community organizers, eliciting and acting on
the needs of the communities they served. With the advent of WtW funding, CHAs were reframed through a series of administrative practices to
become welfare recipients who were in need of "work experience." The
training they received was modified to acculturate them to the "world of

work," while their bodies in the workplace became the "outcomes" that were counted to demonstrate the program's success.

These interventions were justified through appeals to (among other sources) so-called new paternalists such as Lawrence Mead, a major force behind work requirements and U.S. welfare reform policies. They acquired their moniker because of their belief that welfare recipients need *more*, not less, state intervention in their lives to shape them into productive citizens (Schram 2000). Explaining the new paternalist approach, Mead writes, "The final option for antipoverty policy [1996 welfare reform] represents a return to a citizenship rationale, but this time with the emphasis on obligations rather than rights. The argument is that, if nonwork and other incivilities have weakened the welfare state, then work and other duties should be enforced" (Lawrence Mead, qtd. in Schram 2000, 36).

Throughout, the gendered nature of CHAs' work both in the community as health advocates and as welfare recipients remained implicit. Seldom if ever did I hear CHA trainers or program coordinators discuss CHAs' roles *as* women; women's role as the family member responsible for health care or for ensuring that their kids got their shots remained completely naturalized. Program coordinators and trainers even sought to capitalize on the "natural" association of women, especially poor women, with children and family responsibilities by encouraging CHAs to "bond" with the families in their target neighborhoods by sharing stories about parenting their own children (see Gupta and Sharma 2006). In her analysis of the complex relations among concepts of community, identity, and nation, Miranda Joseph points to the centrality of gender to processes of community and national development, cautioning against naturalized ideas of authenticity built on gendered ideals. She observes, "Feminist theorists of both Northern and Southern nationalisms have argued that the articulation of national collectivities often depends on the regulation of gender and the control of women, even as women emerge as privileged bearers of 'culture' and 'community.' These arguments suggest that in taking up communitarian nationalist discourse as a discourse of emancipation, of autonomy and authenticity, both Marxist and liberal postcolonial nationalisms have inscribed oppression into their own practices" (2002, xx). As a technology of governing, the CHA program seamlessly, almost invisibly, incorporated stereotypes about reproduction and welfare dependency into its gendered assumptions about women's roles in the family and community. It is noteworthy that the kinds of feminist critiques summarized by Joseph did not seem to enter into Mercedes Cota's or Niara Kadar's responses to WtW funding with their firmly grounded political-economic critiques, however.

Both models of citizenship (community health and WtW) justified their existence by appealing to the good of the larger community. Not only would individuals be empowered and/or employed, but the larger population would also see improvement as a result. The empowerment model called this effect "increased *community capacity*" (Minkler and Wallerstein 1997). In addition, both the community health and WtW approaches constructed poor communities in general, and welfare recipients in particular, as in need, while offering their distinct solutions. Both programs maintained some level of pragmatic assistance for individual health advocates by offering transportation, child care, and so on. Both relied on these supportive services *in order to* secure participation by welfare recipients. Both versions of the CHA program were limited by funding parameters to conducting certain kinds of activities. While their rhetoric and worldviews clearly differed, it is their mutual ability to function as techniques of government that are examined here. Techniques of government are not about the application of power to subjects for the purposes of domination; rather, they seek to enroll and mobilize citizen-subjects in the project of governing, because liberal government requires the active participation and consent of those who are governed (Reed-Danahay and Brettell 2008).[20]

Technologies of citizenship, however, can and do serve multiple ends. What is particularly interesting about the transitions I witnessed in the CHA program is the way that particular keywords or concepts served as focal points for each approach to governing the poor. The same concepts were mobilized by both, with broadly differing consequences in terms of the role of government in the lives of the poor.[21] The remainder of this chapter focuses on three aspects of the CHA program that highlight the transitions and overlaps between the two moments of its development— empowerment, personal responsibility, and participation. I examine these key concepts as nodes of language and practice that reveal the relationships of governance active in the CHA program.

If you asked Mercedes Cota what the ultimate goal of the CHA program was when she helped design it, she would answer, "empowerment." This concept was omnipresent in the CHA training programs I observed and was a central part of the philosophy of this and many other CHA programs.[22] Empowerment meant "enabling people to live their potential." Empowerment was also a way of relating to individual clients, or as Cota put it, "doing things *with* people rather than doing things *for* people."

---

20. "[Techniques of government] frequently require and integrate within them ways in which individuals conduct themselves. That is to say, they involve governed individuals adopting particular practical relations to themselves in the exercise of their freedom in appropriate ways" (Burchell 1996, 36).
21. And here my analysis diverges from that of Akhil Gupta and Aradhana Sharma (2006), who track the similarities in outcomes between two programs for women in India; they find that both liberal welfare assistance and neoliberal empowerment programs are subject to the same forces of transnational governance and development, with similar effects on those served. Here I explore the coexistence of two ideologies of governing in one program and the divergent outcomes of these ideologies.
22. See, for example, Meister et al. 1992, Parker et al. 1998, and Thompson et al. 1999.

Translated to the individual level, this language of empowerment becomes *self-sufficiency*, a value that is visible throughout welfare reform and in myriad other social programs (Clarke 2007). What meanings and capacities does the term *empowerment* carry that render it usable by those who would support no other aspect of Cota's and Kadar's training program for CHAs? Both empowerment and self-sufficiency produce a subject that is independent and capable (Lyon-Callo 2004). A self-sufficient subject is productive, able to support her family without assistance (unless it's from her husband, for then they are enacting "family values"), educates herself to earn a living wage, and engages in the consumer marketplace.[23] An empowered subject is one who is self-determining as well as self-supporting, and, further, committed to fostering the empowerment of others. The discourse of self-sufficiency as deployed in welfare reform rhetoric to describe women on welfare clearly replaces gendered stereotypes of dependency with masculinist norms of independence. Interestingly, the possible gendered parallels in discourses of empowerment, especially as they were mobilized with regard to women of color, were seldom if ever remarked upon in the CHA training.

CHAs' roles in taking care of the people they served (akin to the pastoral relationship of social workers described earlier) conflicted with their aim to "empower" community members to "help themselves." Charo Rodriguez, a CHA in Brighton Square, told a story about a family she had befriended as a CHA. The family often appeared at her office to ask for help translating things such as driver's license applications. In the training, Cota responded, "You have to encourage them to do it themselves." The downside of establishing trusting relationships with community members lay in the possibility that their clients might turn to them too often for help, and CHAs were warned against "doing for" people things they could do for themselves. While it was acceptable to provide help with phone calls and forms, Cota and Kadar told the CHAs to always try to show people how to do it themselves, even if this meant only showing them other places to go for help.

The instability of this relationship of caring and empowering was reflected in the language CHAs used to talk about their work with the people-who-are-not-clients. Trainers referred to them as "the people we serve"—CHAs and trainers alike saw themselves as helping or *serving* neighborhood residents. But when CHAs used the term they often made the noun into a verb, saying, "we *service* the community" or "the people we service." This expression emphasized both the consumer-transaction

---

23. Others have explored marriage promotion in welfare reform as a contemporary technique to reestablish patriarchal family norms and a response to cultural anxieties around sexuality and kinship; see, for example, Duggan 2004; Heath 2009; Polikoff 2008; Scott, London, and Gross 2007; Smith 2007; and Joseph 2002, 92.

aspect of their contact with neighborhood residents, in the sense of "customer service," and the CHAs' embeddedness within a social service context. One of a CHA's main functions was to expand access to locally available services by bringing word of programs to people's doors. When CHAs were revising their résumés after completing their twenty-six weeks of work in the WtW program, Nikki Sparrow, TCHC's program coordinator, suggested the phrase *customer service* as a more generally understood description of the work they did as CHAs. These beliefs about the work CHAs do, and the kind of relations they might establish with people, reveal the range of positionings available to CHAs—and the complex directionality of this particular meaning of *empowerment*.

Under WtW, the CHA program's goal of community empowerment was recycled and regenerated as a synonym for productive citizenry and appropriate consumption. WtW policies defined empowerment *individually* and *economically*. Welfare reform is supposed to produce individualized subjects who are *self-sufficient* and not dependent on "handouts" from the state. Self-sufficiency also signifies the rights and responsibilities of citizenship (Schram 2000), and its incorporation of active citizenship allows left liberals to use the language of self-sufficiency to express their views about the failings of the welfare state in terms that are more acceptable to conservatives and neoliberals. At the same time, the language of community empowerment is used to justify changes in the structure and administration of welfare by policy makers and legislators who draw on the "rhetoric of community development, with empowerment and partnership as central organising principles . . . to facilitate these changes" (Miller and Ahmad 1997, 274). In an in-depth interview with Niara Kadar, I tried to explore the complex and even divergent implications of the term *community capacity building*, which often accompanies terms such as *empowerment* and *participation* in public health literature.[24] Over soup and salads at the local Spaghetti Factory, we talked about politicians' use of the catchphrase to indicate shrinking government resources. *Community capacity* extends meanings of *self-sufficiency* from individuals to communities. Its primary meaning is the ability of communities to identify and solve problems by mobilizing resources. In her comments, Kadar understands the flight of resources that accompanies neoliberalism and globalization in terms of

---

24. *Community capacity* became a keyword in public health starting in the late 1990s. Its synonyms include *community problem-solving ability, community organization*, and *community development*. Community capacity was the opposite of dependency, poverty, disorganization, and violence. In the late 1990s, "community capacity-building" was a difficult-to-quantify but oft-repeated goal of a range of public health programs. For example, the Kellogg Foundation–funded Community Based Public Health Initiative aimed to "increase community capacity" by fostering partnerships between schools of public health and local communities. See Goodman et al. 1998 and Israel et al. 1998 for examples.

citizenship, describing a sense of abandoned, and burdened, urban communities:

> On the one hand, it feels as though people are throwing the weight of this new shift in the way government and business are functioning in society onto the communities. It's now saying to folks, "Well, we got our own fish to fry over here. We're no longer interested in domestic issues. The government's pulling out and taking a lot of their resources with them as they go, and then, on the other hand, businesses are not putting their dollars in their communities anymore or putting infrastructure in the community because they're over there building an entire factory." So now all of a sudden here we are as communities faced with these major, major issues. In communities where previously we felt there was a governmental responsibility, people now suddenly are coming up with this new social, civic responsibility. And because you're now having to address [the question] where is the citizen, and where is the community, and where are we as collaboratives and concerned people now going to fill in where others historically have done this for us? For the last decade in this society we have been able to look to the government . . . for support around these issues, and they're withdrawing. So these phrases have begun to jump up—this whole business of capacity building, civic responsibility, democracy in action—all these little catchphrases that now say to you and me, you know, they're out of here, so what the hell are we going to do now with folks dying all around us, and folks becoming more homeless, and babies more hungry, and women without support or income, and men leaving their families—what are we going to do?

Her response is to assert a specific vision of collaborative capacity building that is egalitarian in cause and effect, that does not disproportionately place responsibility on poor and minority communities:

> I guess from my perspective as long as the capacity-building issues are not strictly the responsibility of the community, as long as we talk capacity building across all segments—as long as we're saying, yes, every corporation in this community has to come together; yes, all the forces of police, municipal government, the school; yes, the citizen's groups; yes, the minority community agencies; yes, those other agencies   as long as all those folks are able to sit down and say, "How do we pool resources and address these issues to become people's mutual issues on a community level," fine. But if you're going to just throw that capacity building into the Latino community in [Brighton Square] and say, okay, these are your issues,

HIV/AIDS is your issue, look to the state to get a few bucks but that basically whatever you've got internally, you're gonna have to use—you're in trouble. We're in big trouble.

Here I noted that Cota frequently used the term *community capacity* in a positive sense, as a goal of the CHA program, to see how Kadar would explain its other meaning:

> Susan: That seems very descriptive. . . . So what's on the good side of capacity building?
>
> Niara: I think when [Mercedes] speaks of capacity building, my sense of her approach to this would be that, essentially, all good movements have come from grass roots. Anything of any significance has come from the grass roots first—that, in fact, you can expect the oppressed to solve the problems that the oppressors cause. . . . But people have to have some ability to be able to understand how to do that. Now when I think of the civil rights movement, the civil rights movement wasn't started by Martin Luther King or Rosa Parks. The civil rights movements really happened from students who came together around issues that they decided that they were going to begin to address. And because [of] the power of the students and working in these communities, the leadership of the organized black church moved in on that. That didn't come from them. And they began the movement in black churches. Okay? . . . Martin Luther King came in after the fact; he certainly was a boon and a benefit overall, but, I mean, the bottom line was it wasn't his idea.
>
> So where I think she [Mercedes] comes from a lot of the time when she talks about capacity building, she talks about grass-roots organizing. And I think that's where she always wants the CHAs to go and what she wants them to do. Not just tools of the establishment [*laughs*] but the actual grassroots organizers, who are like union workers in the trade unions, and others like those, who actually went in and began to organize the people and because they did that, things happened and came from the people. So that's the good side of capacity building.

In this set of reflections, CHA trainer Niara Kadar articulates the double-edged, ambivalent meanings of the concept of "community capacity building" that mirror the possibilities of self-sufficiency and personal responsibility. Neoliberal social programs seek to increase community capacity as part of the transfer of responsibility for social welfare from the state to community or private NGOs. Community health activists like Cota and Kadar are interested in promoting community capacity as a type of grassroots community mobilization. Here Kadar renarrates social movement history in a way that invokes the complex and unstable meanings of insider/outsider as she highlights the role of student activists over that of Dr. Martin Luther King, Jr., in the civil rights movement. While, for some, community organizing depends on a certain politics of authenticity and representation, the history Kadar produces here presents a messy and layered understanding of community transformation in which engagement and effectiveness seem to trump categories of authenticity, purity, or belonging (Joseph 2002). The prevalence of discussions about "community capacity building" during a time of neoliberal retrenchment speaks to the way that community participation is mobilized in neoliberal government, which governs citizens by encouraging them to act on their interests insofar as those are constructed as consonant with those of the state.[25]

Community Participation: The Reintegration of Communities as Subjects of Government

The community empowerment model also sought participation from members of the larger community, for example, by attending health education workshops, signing up for health insurance, or taking part in community organizing efforts. After Massachusetts's welfare reform, work programs were mandatory, yet frequently described as though recipients exercised free choice to take part. WtW programs face the same challenges as community health organizations, however, in "eliciting" the participation of the target population (Riccio and Hasenfeld 1996). Similarly, in the field of community health, the notion of empowerment is closely tied up with the concept of community participation (Little 2009; Gastaldo 1997, 124).[26] In their trainings for the CHAs, Cota and Kadar constantly stressed how important it was for community members to be involved in different aspects of the CHA program.[27] Several different layers of participation made up the CHAs' work, from signing people up for health insurance

---

25. Andrew Metcalfe (1993, 40) has a particularly incisive critique for this approach. He writes that health promotion programs "offer to produce people who share the values of the dominant class, who monitor their own adherence to these values, and who are therefore likely to seek purely personal solutions to truly social problems."

26. Michael Marinetto (2003) provides a review of the role of the state in mobilization, defining and shaping practices of "community involvement" in twenty years of British programs seeking greater participation in local government.

27. Cota and Kadar practiced what Denise Gastaldo would call "radical health education," as they were "committed to combating social inequality in a broad way and [to] promoting community participation in health issues" (1997, 117). Gastaldo contrasts this with "traditional health education," an approach that "concentrate[s] on individuals' responsibility for health and disease prevention" (1997, 117).

to attending health education workshops, each of which placed the community member in a relationship of governance with the health advocate. CHAs struggled with their roles as community change agents and as agents of the state, finding themselves pushed by accounting requirements to document outcomes such as number of families enrolled in health insurance and pulled by the desire to help others.

Just as community health education programs rely on a range of strategies to "elicit participation," so do welfare programs. A large policy literature in social work and public policy is devoted to the question of participation in voluntary work programs. Persuading people on welfare to actually take part in these programs has led to all sorts of innovations from program planners. Often, however, as in the CHA program, this participation is more fictive than real. One team of policy researchers writes, "Participation in the work and training program was offered not as a route to self-sufficiency but as a compliance requirement for staying on welfare—much like bringing in a rent receipt or a utility bill" (Bane and Ellwood 1994, 6). Though Massachusetts welfare reform now relies on work mandates rather than voluntary programs, the same challenges to participation still present themselves in Thornton's welfare offices.

The social work literature is frank about the slippery slope between participation and coercion: "Critics of participation requirements have argued that . . . eliciting the desired forms of compliance (e.g., participation in assigned employment-related activities) through 'coercion' can be administratively difficult and at cross-purposes with building an organizational culture that stresses enthusiasm for work . . ." (Riccio and Hasenfeld 1996, 517). Writing in the *Social Service Review*, James Riccio and Yeheskel Hasenfeld discuss three strategies for getting people on welfare to participate in work programs: constraints, inducements, and persuasion. After serious consideration, the authors conclude that persuasion is a better choice for inducing participation than are constraints, because constraints encourage evasion and require "continuous surveillance of clients' behavior." Persuasion, in contrast, encourages self-governing subjects: persuasion "is considered more likely to produce enduring behavioral changes because the desired values and beliefs are internalized and do not require monitoring" (Riccio and Hasenfeld 1996, 521). In other words, participatory practices are more effective because they are more efficient; this form of shaping the conduct of conduct (Foucault 1991) requires less work on the part of those who govern to monitor those who are governed. Further, the "will to participate" is located within, called forth from, an existing structure governed by the demands of profit, sustainability, and so on. It follows, then, that the programmatic solution for "dependent" subjects is not (simply) more services, but rather their engagement as active citizens through practices of community participation and participatory education.

Each of the three concepts discussed here—empowerment, self-sufficiency, and participation—functions as a point of intersection for two different models of governing the poor: the community health approach outlined in Chapter 2 and the WtW approach presented here. To highlight the differences between the approaches, I discuss the specific meanings and inflections of these nodes of language and practice (e.g., the kinds of citizens that are being created; the kind of community that is envisioned). Both approaches, however, shared some capacities as techniques of government. Techniques of community empowerment and job training programs attempt to shape the conduct of people on welfare, as well as those who govern them. At the same time, the concepts, terms, and practices that emerge from their divergent political genealogies retained their different meanings in practice—for example, the importance of forming a group identity among CHAs in the community empowerment model. Insofar as these nodes share the ability to describe relations of government, they are available for use by neoliberal policy makers (Lyon-Callo 2004). But we cannot speak simply of the "appropriation" of the language of empowerment by the political right. Advocates for neoliberal reforms have been able to mobilize the language of the left in justifying the devolution and privatization of services. An emphasis on an independent and self-governing subject, for example, and a vision of self-improvement for subjects previously defined by their marginalization render the language of empowerment suitable for use by those who describe a very different political vision from that of community health activists (Cruikshank 1999; Dean 1999). Both the community health and WtW approaches result from different attempts to answer the question: What is needed, and what is good, in the government of "our" cities and communities? Notions of participation and representation are of special interest as various groups negotiate new forms of government in the post-welfare state.

Concepts of empowerment and community capacity building crystallize discourses and practices concerned with the identity and conduct of the poor. In fact, the local, dispersed, yet publicly supported (through welfare reform) community organizers imagined in the CHA program exemplify postmodern governance as nonstate actors serve state goals such as improving the public health. In the community empowerment model, CHAs are envisioned as ideal citizens mobilized on the basis of their roles as family members responsible for community health. The implicit work of gender helps construct African American and Latina women as the best suited to reach their target populations. Health advocates here are being trained as agents of government whose task (if they fully adopt their trainers' "analysis of oppression") is, in a certain respect, to undermine the oppressive practices of the existing government. In contrast, the goal of the WtW model is to transform dependent welfare mothers into self-sufficient citizens. However, despite the language of community uplift, welfare reform policies hampered the involvement of those most likely to engage in the process of community empowerment by designating a new population, the "hardest to serve," and assigning funding to the group least likely or able to take part. In seeking to refashion women on welfare as productive citizens who are willing and able to insert themselves into the service economy, welfare reform created more obstacles than doorways to economic participation. The "work first" approach disallows important requisites for employment for those designated "hardest to serve," such as publicly funded drug treatment or education. Thus the only avenues created by WtW for community capacity building is individualized employment in low-wage, unskilled jobs in which employers take the place of welfare workers, yet with no obligation for retention or promotion.

The expansion of economic rationalities through the nonprofit sector is not yet complete, however. I saw much on-the-ground conflict among local organizations who would go far to resist such changes in their programs. Their struggles illustrate that while the notion of *community* increasingly serves as a terrain of government, its meanings are still contested, and countering visions still enliven the work of many who see themselves as working in the trenches of social welfare. This and other sites of contestation provide nuanced examples of the unintended effects of community mobilizing for change. Chapter 4 turns our attention to other means by which health care providers seek to manage the problem of cultural differences in health care.

4

Technologies of Culturally Appropriate Health Care

In the mid-1990s in Thornton, Massachusetts, activists and community health leaders worked to establish what would become Thornton Community Health Center (TCHC) as part of a struggle to bring quality, culturally appropriate health care to low-income and minority patients. According to organizers, economically and ethnically marginalized Thornton residents were unable to obtain quality care from existing health care resources (Shaw 2005). When I began my fieldwork there in 1998, TCHC had been caring for patients for two years but still struggled with the best way to reach so-called hard-to-serve residents of its surrounding neighborhoods. Building on established models of lay health advisors (Eng, Parker, and Harlan 1997), the Community Health Advocate (CHA) program described in previous chapters mobilized local residents as outreach workers to bring medically underserved residents into the clinic. Once they arrived, however, ethnic, cultural, and linguistic differences between these new patients and TCHC's staff and health care providers remained an issue, as the clinic struggled to locate medical interpreters or when a patient complained about prejudicial behavior from a physician. George Williams, executive director of TCHC for its first nine years, therefore maintained an active interest in culturally appropriate health care—efforts to tailor health care to the distinctive needs of different cultural groups (Shaw 2005). For example, Williams created a standing committee tasked with designing policies and procedures to foster culturally appropriate health care, and the clinic underwent an organizational cultural competence assessment by researchers at Georgetown University.

Observing this process prompted me to subscribe to an e-mail discussion list (which I here call the Culture and Health list) where health care administrators, medical interpreters, and other cultural competence (CC) experts use e-mail to share resources and information in a collective yet dispersed effort to address the effects of cultural difference in the clinic. This chapter draws on five years of postings to the Culture and Health list, as well as on participant-observation research at conferences attended by health care administrators and CC trainers, to discover how culturally appropriate health care has emerged as another widely promoted remedy to the same problems of cultural difference that the CHA program, in its inception, sought to overcome. I explore culturally appropriate health care as a novel formation encompassing both face-to-face and electronic technologies that contributes to the development and dissemination of new forms of expertise in health care. Much of the ethnography on which this chapter is based comes not from a particular clinical setting but rather forums such as the Culture and Health list where participants from all over the world discuss topics of culture and health care.

I explore the processes through which cultural expertise is being developed, codified, and disseminated through analyses of five years of postings to this moderated e-mail list. The Culture and Health list has nearly two thousand members at last count and is sponsored by an international nonprofit organization that claims a central role in the development of the CLAS regulations and holds a biannual conference that I attended in 2008. Those who post to the list, whom I refer to as posters, include health care administrators, medical interpreters, anthropologists, and cultural competence experts and trainers. Subscribers tend to be those who have been assigned responsibility for ensuring compliance with the CLAS regulations or for handling issues related to cultural diversity in their health care organizations (e.g., diversity officers or directors of medical interpreter departments). While a wide range of e-mail lists, blogs, and Web sites feed the public appetite for information on topics related to culture and health, the Culture and Health list fills a special niche. A forum for the exchange of information (often in the form of links to other Web pages), views, and opinions, the Culture and Health list helps establish and disseminate cultural expertise—both as a group and as individuals—and actively creates a shared, if contested, narrative (Mattingly 1998) about cultural competence programs.[1] This chapter traces the emergence of cultural competency as a

---

1. I was an unannounced "lurker" on this list. As noted previously, all names and identifying features have been changed to maintain anonymity, but it is worth noting that current guidelines indicate that the consensus among scholars is that e-mails to this sort of list are public and therefore not subject to narrower privacy concerns (see Ess and the Association of Internet Researchers 2002).

discourse of technical expertise by analyzing texts that reveal contestations over the parameters of cultural expertise and the meaning and regulation of difference in health care. I explore arenas of struggle among stakeholders who strive to balance the perceived efficacy of modularized forms of knowledge with calls for individualized, patient-centered care.

Health Disparities and Culturally Appropriate Health Care

Preceded by related efforts such as patient-centered health care (Laine and Davidoff 1996), the social formation now known as culturally appropriate health care crystallized in response to reports of ethnic disparities in health status and quality of care that emerged as critiques of social inequality in the United States (Shaw 2005; Institute of Medicine et al. 2003; Epstein 2007). Advocacy groups use health statistics revealing patterned inequalities among racial and ethnic minority groups to demand recognition and resources from the state (Santiago-Irizarry 2001; Wailoo 2001), to contest medical expertise (Hogle 2002a), and to seek changes to make primary health care more "culturally appropriate" (L. Anderson et al. 2003). Political claims for equality of access, or separate "culturally appropriate" programs for minority groups, are based on an appeal for recognition of the unique cultural features, experiences, or history of oppression of a given group (Santiago-Irizarry 2001), naturalizing the cultural identity of white people in the process. The practical consequences of this politics of recognition (Fraser 2001) for health care may range from new hospital gowns to medical interpreters to larger exam rooms that more easily accommodate extended families. These and other innovations make up *culturally appropriate health care*, which is often proposed as a remedy for health disparities, particularly those associated with health care quality and discrimination.[2]

As minority advocacy groups and others seek to make health care more inclusive for diverse populations, new interventions are being developed to address barriers of access and incommensurability, expanding the regimes of knowledge that are available to health care providers.[3] An emerging "cultural competence" industry generates and distributes specialized social expertise to teach health care providers how best to respond to "cultural difference" in clinical encounters. Technologies of culturally appropriate

---

2. For anthropological investigations of elements of this process, see Borovoy and Hine 2008; Jenks 2009; Ong 1995; Sargent and Larchanché 2009; Taylor 2003b; Willen, Bullen, and Good 2010; Good et al. 2011; and Mattingly 2006. Others have addressed this topic and related or narrower aspects of it using the terms *cultural competence, cultural sensitivity, cultural awareness*, and *cultural humility*, among others. For reviews of this voluminous literature in medicine and public health, see Beach et al. 2005; L. Anderson et al. 2003; Kehoe, Melkus, and Newlin 2003; and Manson 2003.

3. See Epstein 2007 for a cultural analysis of similar moves in biomedical research.

According to the CLAS guidelines, health care organizations should

1. Ensure that care is "provided in a manner compatible with the cultural health beliefs and practices and preferred language" of patients.
2. Recruit, retain, and promote a diverse and representative staff.
3. Ensure that all staff receive ongoing education in cultural competence.
4. Provide language-assistance services to patients at no cost.
5. Provide verbal offers and written notices in patients' preferred language informing them of their right to receive language-assistance services.
6. Ensure the competence of language assistance and avoid using family members as translators.
7. Post signage in all languages.
8. Develop a strategic plan for implementing CLAS.
9. Conduct organizational self-assessments.
10. Collect racial, ethnic, and language data on patients. . . .
12. Develop collaborative partnerships with communities to facilitate patient involvement.
13. Develop culturally sensitive conflict-resolution procedures.
14. Publicize innovations involving CLAS.

Only items 4 through 7 are *mandates*, current federal requirements for all recipients of federal funds. CLAS *guidelines* (items 1 through 3 and 8 through 13) have been recommended by OMH for adoption as mandates. *Recommendations* (item 14) are suggested by OMH for voluntary adoption by health care organizations.

Source: U.S. Department of Health and Human Services 2007.

The Culturally and Linguistically Appropriate Services (CLAS) guidelines.

health care are designed to produce more equal health outcomes by eliminating prejudice among health care providers and reducing disparities in patient care across groups.[4] In so doing, technologies of culturally appro-

---

4. Another approach to eliminating disparities in quality of health care is through workforce diversity programs. These initiatives promote the recruitment of more minority health care providers to increase access to and quality of health care for medically underserved and minority patients (Shaw 2010). Yet the distribution of access to medical professions

priate health care govern the conduct of both medical professionals and patients as they produce not only new kinds of ethical, self-reflexive medical professionals but also new kinds of "culturally diverse," "immigrant," "refugee," and "minority" patients as well.

Culturally appropriate health care is becoming increasingly tightly integrated in both public and private regulatory regimes. In a first step, in response to calls from minority groups for policy solutions to health disparities, the U.S. Office of Minority Health proposed regulations in 2001 requiring health care providers and organizations who receive federal funds to provide "culturally and linguistically appropriate services" (CLAS). More recently, elements of these regulations have been adopted by the Joint Commission, the hospital accreditation agency, in its annual survey.[5] Yet the knowledge and practices that constitute the discursive formation that is culturally appropriate health care are not as monolithic as might be construed based on a superficial reading of these developments. Indeed, culturally appropriate health care (CAHC) is made up of variable and at times contradictory practices, pushed forward by aims that range from antiracist immigrants' rights efforts to health care quality improvement initiatives.

Emerging Cultural Expertise

Cultural competency programs for health care providers function as new social technologies that develop and transfer cultural expertise in order to modify doctor-patient interactions to address ethnic and cultural disparities in medical practice. Diversity trainers, medical anthropologists, and other professionals contribute to the formation of specialized social expertise that is disseminated through programs designed to teach health care providers how best to respond to "difference" in clinical encounters. The CLAS regulations and their integration into Joint Commission accreditation standards create new opportunities for these holders of marginalized forms of expertise in health care to consolidate their knowledge and increase its legitimacy. My analysis builds on Nikolas Rose's understanding of expertise as "a particular kind of social *authority*, grounded in a claim to *truth*, asserting technical *efficacy*, and avowing *humane* ethical virtues" (Rose 1998, 86). Claims for the recognition of difference in health care are seen by some as undermining and fracturing universalizing biomedical

---

in the United States continues to ensure that health care providers are disproportionately white and privileged (Sullivan and Mittman 2010; Steinecke and Terrell 2010).

5. A private nonprofit organization, the Joint Commission is often known by its former name, the Joint Commission on Accreditation of Healthcare Organizations, or JCAHO (pronounced "jay-co"). While accreditation is voluntary, it is linked to insurance reimbursement and thus its mandates and guidelines have the force of law (or, absent legal sanctions, even greater force).

expertise into myriad population-specific parts (Hannah 2008). The developments described here are "partial and provisional reconfigurations of 'ethical' reflection and action" (Ong and Collier 2005, 30) by those who seek to modify health care to recognize, accommodate, and respond to cultural differences among patients, and between patients and health care providers. CAHC advocates compete with other knowledge specialists as they try to integrate cultural competence into current economic structures of health care (Anderson, Tang, and Blue 2007). These new "cultural experts" are creating and disseminating the authority of their expertise using shared curricula, standards, policies, and procedures that "avow the *humane* ethical virtues" of equality and justice in health care.

For many health care providers, the expertise of culture may ultimately aid their competitive struggle for position brought on by shrinking reimbursements and recession. As Marit Melhuus observes, "Culture is good business, as it is good politics: it works well, or so it has seemed" (1999, 68). In their study of ethnicity and the commodification of culture, anthropologists John and Jean Comaroff argue that ethnic identity is both produced and consumed through practices and discourses that circulate through globalized nationalities (Comaroff and Comaroff 2009). Here I trace the process of translating the expertise of culture into terms that biomedical providers and health care administrators can understand as valid and persuasive.

As part of the project to manage difference more efficiently in the clinic, health care providers are called on to reorient their practice (habits of gaze, touch, decision making) and to act on their own subjectivities in order to become "culturally competent." Health care providers, not patients, are thus the subjects of cultural competence training. Diversity trainers, antiracism and social justice activists, medical anthropologists, and other CC program designers disseminate specialized forms of expertise designed to teach health care providers how best to respond to "difference" in clinical encounters. List members exchange information, queries, views, and advice on the standardized forms of knowledge that proliferate around cultural competence "interventions" for health care providers. Requests for standardized knowledge take many different forms; for example, a poster may ask for "recommendations for or key opinion leaders (clinicians) re: cultural competence when managing HIV/AIDS in the Hispanic population." Another poster requested guides for culturally appropriate touch between health care providers and members of different cultural groups; and another sought a "diversity and culture learning needs assessment for pediatric hospital staff."

New forms of cultural expertise are being produced and circulated in domains such as the Culture and Health list and in face-to-face cultural competence trainings. These bodies of knowledge must be squeezed into existing conventions of instrumental rationality (e.g., Collier and Ong

2005). As the CLAS regulations filter down from hospitals and health care providers to the level of community organizations, well-intentioned workers are tasked with the need to assess their own cultural competence and that of their organization, and then to locate a means to increase it. This was evident in a request for training resources posted to the Culture and Health list by a Catholic social service agency staff member, who outlined the features of CC interventions that administrators like her would find desirable:

> Something web-based with modules for different levels of staff that is not expensive to use or purchase would be very helpful. And if you were to expand it beyond the medical system to include mental health, for example, it would be even more helpful. [M]ost of the resources I have been able to find are targeted to health providers and health systems, and the need is much broader than that. My organization is expected to have a "cultural competence plan" to improve our levels of cultural competence. In doing some research to determine what "cultural competence" looks like (in any sort of measurable fashion so that I can develop a plan and a training program to increase it, therefore) has been a challenge. Any assistance in that area would be welcome in my book, and the more concrete the assistance the better!

This administrator's query exemplifies the effects of new forms of governance on the workers on the ground. She responded to the imperative for constant self-assessment and ongoing action on one's own expertise to increase and expand it (Geary 2007)—a key feature of "the transformation of the subjectivity of the worker" (Rose 1999, 162) in answer to the need for permanent reskilling in a continually changing economy.

This process has specifically ethical dimensions in health care, as advocates seek to distribute health care more equitably and improve its quality by remaking health care practice. One poster, for example, articulated the call for CAHC as an ethic of "'diffidence' (or humility)," relocating this ethic within the canon of Hippocratic medicine. Interestingly, in the same paragraph, the poster linked this canon with "the modern QI [Quality Improvement] movement," an effort to control health care costs, eliminate unnecessary care, and improve outcomes by tracking a range of quality indicators in care (Jencks and Wilensky 1992; Scally and Donaldson 1998), via "Percival, Bond, . . . and other forefathers":

> As an historical side-note, the notion of "diffidence" (or humility) as a core value in medicine more generally dates to the Hippocratic era and perhaps earlier—recall, for example, the famous Hippocratic dictum, "Life is short, the art is long, opportunity fleeting,

experiment perilous, judgment difficult." Humility in practice was certainly very prevalent in the writing of John Gregory, who gave the first known set of lectures on medical ethics to medical students in the 1700s; and it is a continuous theme for Percival, Bond, Codman, and many other forefathers of the modern QI movement. Sadly, of course, we doctors haven't always lived up to the ethical ideal of practicing with humility.

Technologies of culturally appropriate health care organize diverse and unpredictable groups of people into categories and populations more easily understood by (implicitly culturally homogeneous) health care providers. CAHC may allow health care providers to diagnose and cure patients more efficiently through prescribed behaviors and information for use with particular populations. Like the population-based health care techniques described previously, CAHC renders populations legible to health care providers and the state by enumerating features of "cultural difference" and providing a bridge for the gaps imposed by incommensurability. In so doing, technologies of CAHC reinscribe older forms of exclusion as the characteristics and traits of difference become reified in handbooks, manuals, and trainings.[6]

On Technologies of Culturally Appropriate Health Care

A variety of techniques have been developed to inculcate health care providers with new information and attitudes toward diverse groups. The ethical health care provider presented in these trainings is one who recognizes racist or prejudicial thoughts in herself and seeks to expunge or at least master them; who understands and accepts the impact of cultural differences on health; who is respectful of patient autonomy and practices patient-centered care; and one who is able to situate each patient in his or her social and cultural context. A plethora of curricula, tools, videos, bibliographies, vignettes, and other resources on cultural competence can be found online. Individual researchers, health care providers, and cultural competence instructors all draw from online resources in searching for information and creating new tools. While online curricula and training activities allow health care providers to engage in training outside the boundaries of the reimbursable workday, many trainers endorse face-to-face training in large

---

6. While many cultural competence trainings contain careful discussions of the difference between generalizations and stereotypes and offer vivid examples of the hazards of making assumptions about individuals on the basis of their supposed "cultural traits," many people both within and outside the emergent field of CAHC express concern regarding the broader effects of the generation and dissemination of these regimes of knowledge and practice (e.g., Hannah 2008; Willen, Bullon, and Good 2010; Jenks 2009, 2011; Taylor 2003a).

or small groups as more likely to effect the sought-after transformations of consciousness. For example, Rafael Gonzalez, an instructor who taught an eight-week seminar in cultural competence at a large medical school, explained to me in an in-depth interview:

> Rafael: I've used different venues; I mean I've done it in a small group—"done it," meaning lectured on cultural competency— I've done it online, where I'm videotaped and I'm looking at a screen and there's people out, you know, at different satellite places, you know, [where] there's a monitor. That doesn't work that well, I don't think. Umm . . .
>
> Interviewer: Is that because you don't have the kind of give and take?
>
> Rafael: Don't have that pers—yeah, that interpersonal interaction there, those warm bodies right there in front of you. Umm, plus [it's] more sterile. I think the ideal way is a small-group discussion [where] people are free to talk about their own experiences and then reframe those experiences in terms of what goes on, the reality of the patient-provider interaction. So at one level, one can talk about the patient-provider interaction, which is primarily the case in the College of Medicine. And on another level, you can talk about it as a general approach to community health.

Gonzalez called on the face-to-face experience of the small-group setting as that which offers the most effective technology for accomplishing self-examination by encouraging medical students to "reframe [their clinical] experiences." He rejected CC training via video link as "more sterile" in favor of the "warm bodies right there in front of you," acknowledging the contribution those warm bodies make to the chemistry of the transformations he seeks.

In May 2008 I attended another breakfast roundtable on cultural competence, this one at the Cancer, Culture and Literacy conference sponsored by the Moffitt Cancer Center in Florida. Sam Wolfe, the facilitator, introduced himself as someone who regularly conducts trainings for health care providers, medical faculty, and even military medical personnel. He also described his preference for small-group work over online training, arguing that a onetime workshop is often not as effective as small groups that meet regularly over time: "We run twelve week sessions for those health care organizations that will pay for it. And we dread the first of these meetings. There are two common responses among health care providers on the first meeting: (1) 'I'm already culturally competent' and (2) 'Well, it's the patient's fault.' But what you ultimately want to achieve, and you know you have been successful, when you see peers correcting peers."

Wolfe emphasized the relocation of pedagogical responsibility from trainer to participants—"when you see peers correcting peers"—as an index of the successful inculcation of new forms of expertise and norms of behavior among participants.

Another roundtable participant reported that she felt fortunate to have strong leadership support at her hospital, and she asked Wolfe for guidance as she chose among the various modules available online for CC training. Wolfe repeated that he preferred face-to-face training programs that allow interaction and discussion among participants. Another participant made disparaging noises about trainings that "you click through" (making the hand motion of clicking a mouse in the air). Others at the table agreed. Wolfe concurred but said that if that was the only option, he would choose modules that offer testimonials that can engage participants and encourage them to stop and think. He added, "You want to look for opportunities for self-reflection in the module you choose" and suggested that "poignant stories" allow the participant to do a "double-check."

Technologies of cultural competence often seek to foster these abilities by shifting the onus onto the "learner." For example, at the CAHC conference mentioned previously, Margaret, an audience member, described a continuing medical education (CME) program she developed to train physicians to "incorporate cultural and linguistic competency into the diagnosis and treatment of depression." This program began with a self-assessment in which the physician is first asked to rate her own cultural competence using several subscales. Rather than getting a score, Margaret explained, "because, you know, who cares what you score on a cultural competence test," the physician then is able to "self-select" the items that she might want to "promote in her learning." The participant also chooses her preferred medium for the module (e.g., text or video). At the end of the module, the "learner" is matched to a behavioral "action plan based on [her] individual responses to the subscales so that it should be self-motivating." Rather than positioning the physician as the passive recipient of information, which is often less than successful, Margaret's CME program makes the physician responsible for "choosing" not only the content of the training but even the medium in which it is delivered. The link with behavior is accomplished by the individualized "action plan" generated by the program in response to these selections.

Resistance

Many Culture and Health posters recount their efforts to implement the CLAS guidelines in their health care organizations but describe a variety of barriers, including resistance to organizational change or the "outsider" status of cultural expertise. For example, Maria Silva, a language services coordinator for an academic medical center, wrote:

As my Language Services staff continue to struggle with daily refusals on the part of medical/support staff to use the many tools for appropriate language access that we provide, we are wondering if anyone has found a non-threatening/anonymous way to directly ask those staff why they make that choice. We in Language Services have frequent discussions with those staff and know that their answers are generally one of the following: (a) It costs too much. (b) It takes too much time. (c) It isn't necessary—they speak "enough" English. (d) They brought someone with them who speaks English. (e) They don't deserve it—they should learn English. However, our anecdotal information is viewed as suspect by many staff people who want quantifiable proof that people are refusing to use language access tools. Has anyone out there devised a way that would be seen as "evidence based" and backed up with "scientific data" to get staff to give their views on interpreter/translation services and reasons for not using?

Knowledge about cultural differences, along with qualitative data in medicine more generally, is marginalized by virtue of its "softness," its inability to deliver conclusions with p-values, confidence intervals, or a biological mechanism (Taylor 2003a). Medical education and health care institutions are proving to be less than accommodating to these new forms of cultural expertise. For example, an audience member at the CC training roundtable discussed earlier asked the panelists, "I appreciate your comments about [the importance of] teaching cultural competence with medical students, but what do you do with residents and that wonderful group of faculty [*this phrase provoked chuckles around the room*] that aren't 'on-board'? What do you do with them?" Panelist Paul Armstrong agreed, "Yeah, I think it's always a challenge to figure out, how do you reach everyone. I think that one of the approaches we've taken is to figure what the leverage points are for those individuals to be interested in this. What would make them interested in a training around something that we might call 'cultural competency'?" To address this resistance, Armstrong and other CC trainers enwrap CC education in a familiar format, situating their approach firmly in the biomedical case method (see Good and Good 1993):

So we've tried to . . . build in very interactive cases where you'd be challenged to actually think, "what's going on with this patient? I just don't understand it." Clinicians specifically, but everyone really tends to have a drive to solve the problem. That's what we try to build in there. Let's make a problem, and then let's generate their creative, and get their competitive juices flowing, almost, about, "All right, can I figure it out what's going on with this person?"

Then they go through it and in the end wind up hopefully being able to crack the case, solve the problem. And, of course it's not so easy, there's no *one* answer, but they feel as they're going through it that they're trying to get somewhere, and as they go through the process they learn pieces of information along the way.

Similarly, Rafael Gonzalez, the CC instructor introduced previously, perceived significant resistance among the other medical school faculty to integrate cultural competence themes and topics into the medical school curriculum. He felt that while

there was buy-in from the administration and the College of Medicine at that time, there wasn't a whole lot of buy-in from the departmental heads and regular faculty. Basically if you wanted to include anything on culture and linguistic competency, they wanted you to come in and do it yourself and have it stand alone, and they didn't necessarily wanna take up their time in doing that. . . . Basically they felt that . . . they had already had a short amount of time to present the information necessary in the basic science courses. So I tried to facilitate the development of vignettes that we could share to highlight examples of issues that could confront folks—for example, in genetic counseling, umm, and those courses that are more amenable to those kinds of vignettes. But there was resistance, again, primarily time management and . . . the lack of expertise on cultural competency among the professors themselves, and them wanting someone else to do it rather than themselves.

While Gonzalez made a similar effort to offer CC training using "vignettes" tailored to fields such as genetic counseling that he saw as "more amenable" to such interventions, other medical school faculty viewed the whole endeavor as so marginal as to be unworthy of their own time and effort (and barely worthy of that of their students), and as something to be delegated to others.

Modularized Knowledge: Technological Reason and Patient-Centered Health Care

In addition to embedding technologies of CAHC in broader reform efforts such as QI or patient-centered health care, posters on the Culture and Health list actively construct legitimacy for their marginalized forms of knowledge in several ways: through pushing for certification of medical interpreters, for example, or in discussions about how to produce measurable outcomes for cultural competence interventions. Studies of professionalization in other health-related fields show how expert knowledge is constituted through practices of standardization, accreditation, and organized institutions of learning (Cant and Sharma 1996).[7] To achieve widespread legibility for CAHC in health care settings and organizations, list members collaborate in developing and disseminating "modular" knowledge about culture and health, packaged the same way as CME courses. For example, Abigail Kennedy, a public health educator, wrote this request:

> I represent a Medicaid HMO . . . in California. As we are planning staff training, we are looking for a good tool that would help staff identify their unconscious stereotypes. I know of a couple tools which allow medical care staff to self-assess their cultural competence, but our objective here is for health plan staff to have a private way to raise awareness about their biases/racism.
>
> We have experimented with the online [implicit bias] tool at https://implicit.harvard.edu/implicit/. While interesting and revealing, our testers had variable reactions to it.
>
> Do any of you have other suggestions for an online or print tool? Alternatively, a tool for self-assessment of cultural competence that is more oriented to a health plan setting would also be useful.
>
> Note that we have very little budget for this work, so we are seeking something available in the public domain or otherwise without a consultant fee.

This post is emblematic of many aspects of the Culture and Health list. A prepackaged "tool" helps cultural experts disseminate antiracist or cultural education to health care providers quickly and easily, without having to take the time to develop their own curriculum. Though mandated by the state, cultural expertise is not, however, valued enough yet to carry its own line item in organizational budgets, and thus this poster requests a tool that is in the public domain, since so many cultural experts seek to capitalize on their expertise in the for-profit health care environment.[8] The

---

7. The British homeopaths studied by Sarah Cant and Ursula Sharma wish to establish themselves as *competitors* to allopathic medicine, while CAHC trainers seek to increase the legitimacy of their expertise in order to be *accepted and adopted by* biomedical practitioners. CAHC trainers aim to modify the practice of clinical medicine, while homeopaths set themselves as an alternative to clinical medicine (e.g., Cant and Sharma 1996, 582). On professionalization in health care, see also Martin, Currie, and Finn 2009, Hogle 2002b, and Starr 1982.

8. At the 2008 CAHC conference I attended in Minneapolis, Minnesota, which brought together many list members and other public health professionals, the budget as a social and political tool for demonstrating institutional commitment to eliminating health disparities was a constant topic of conversation. Conference participants argued that budgeted funds demonstrated health care organizations' "buy-in," both literal and philosophical, to principles of CAHC, and bemoaned the lack of such line-items. John and Jean Comaroff

bits of modularized knowledge exchanged on the list and in online trainings are designed to be easily consumable and standardized for multiple
users, including administrators, health care providers, and mental health
professionals. Standardized practices are the coin of the realm that allow
modifications of health care practices to be adopted and disseminated in
health care settings, particularly hospitals. The kinds of knowledge that
may be standardized and circulated are diverse, however; posters inquire
about "cultural issues" in asthma management, in "working with caregivers (family/friends) of patients with dementia," or in "palliative care for
'nontraditional populations,'" to name just a few. Online training extends
the wisdom of cultural experts to far-flung areas and overcomes limitations of disciplinary knowledge, space, and time, as health care professionals are able to increase their cultural expertise outside the boundaries
of the reimbursable workday. Indeed, the widespread adoption in cultural
competence circles of the hospitalist language of "universal precautions"
emphasizes the extent to which standardization must be performed by CC
initiatives in order to gain access to these spaces of practice, which depend
on regimentation, accountability, and documentation in the regulation of
flows of patients and profits.

Ambivalent Expertise

Even as posters to the list repeatedly assert and reaffirm the legitimacy of
their cultural expertise, conversation on the Culture and Health list also
reveals a profound ambivalence toward its limits. Amid scores of calls for
tools, measures, and online trainings and resources for health care providers, diversity experts who subscribe to the list interrogate the ethical basis
and possible unintended effects of their implementation. The standardized
forms of knowledge found in cultural competency modules exchanged
and promoted on the list undermine, for some, the ethic of individualized
expertise they advocate. This contradiction forms one of the basic tensions
explored in Part I. The complex politics around the "claims to special
wisdom" that constitute cultural expertise can be glimpsed in the following observation made by Margaret, the diversity trainer and researcher
introduced previously: "When we think about health care, we want our
physicians, nurses, et cetera to be competent. And we don't have an issue
with saying that. But somehow, if it's preceded by the word 'cultural,' we
got all kinds of issues!"

---

discuss the intersections of capital and culture among, in particular, South African ethnic
groups whose identities appear to hinge on the "brand" that is marketed for tourist and
other purposes. They outline the role of market-oriented activity in the production of
subjectivity by means of "*ambiguating* the distinction between producer and consumer,
performer and audience" (2009, 26).

Both within the clinic and beyond its boundaries, interactions around cultural difference are among the aspects of life that are being reorganized by culturally appropriate health care. At the same time that CC advocates exchange bits of modularized knowledge on particular aspects of health and culture, CAHC is often implicitly and occasionally explicitly concerned with recognizing and reforming health care providers' beliefs and practices regarding race, racism, prejudice, and discrimination. The technologies of instrumental reason promoted on the list bump up against a countervailing tendency in CAHC to promote humanistic ideals of equality. For example, in response to a post on "racial quotas" as "(let's admit it) discriminatory practices," Linda McDermott argued, "Privileged people (whites, men, heterosexuals, etc.) have to become conscious of their privilege and understand that it is unjust. That is extremely difficult. It's much easier to cry foul play, injustice and 'reverse discrimination' when 'others' challenge or even seem to challenge that privilege." Subscribers to the list constantly juggle the ethical arguments for changing the conduct of health care by means of new forms of cultural expertise, and the practical circumstances that limit their implementation.

Similar to the ways in which "community" identity becomes the object of work in the CHA trainings described previously, online trainings and face-to-face programs teach health care providers how their patients perform blackness, Latino-ness, and other forms of ethnicity in health care settings. For example, a physician clicking through *The Provider's Guide to Quality and Culture,* a typical online module presented by Management Sciences for Health, may learn that "some Pacific Islanders believe that illness and other misfortune can be attributed to the loss of *mana*, defined as special power or life force. Healing requires the restoration of the imbalance of *mana* through analysis of damaged relationships with one's self, the extended family, ancestors, the environment, or one's spirituality." The NØ STEREOTYPING icons sprinkled throughout the guide's pages are part of the guidance offered to health care providers on how to modify their own attitudes and conduct to best respond to difference in the clinic.[9]

Cultural competence programs promote standardized knowledge to win acceptance by the business of health care, in which best practices and "models" are celebrated for their potential to efficiently improve outcomes. The encroachment of what Stephen Collier and Andrew Lakoff call "technological reason" (2005) in these calls for specialized and standardized knowledge sparked concern for some list members, who experience a conflict with ethical values of cultural relativism and patient-centered care. After reading several requests for modularized information and resources,

---

9. See Management Sciences for Health, n.d. See also Jenks 2011 on the unintended consequences of ongoing efforts in CAHC to deliver cultural content while inoculating health care providers against the tendency to stereotype.

Elizabeth Cooper, a public health nurse, grew frustrated with discussions of what she termed the "fast food"–style delivery of cultural competency and wrote a post that is worth quoting at some length, since it prompted a thoughtful discussion on the list:

> I am increasingly troubled by what I am hearing via email from those who are involved in developing cultural competency programs within their organizations. I feel we are looking for a fast food approach to cultural competency. . . . While I recognize that we have tremendous barriers and upper management that simply does this because it is a mandate, as activists within the field there is a responsibility to continue the message that this is hard work and there are NO quick answers. The idea that cultural competency is achieved through mouse clicks on the internet is at best a joke, and at worst offensive to those of us who day after day engage people of differing cultural values in dialogue about their healthcare. It is not a fast food line where you get it in 5 minutes. It is simultaneously exhausting and rewarding and at the end of the day it is the right thing to do. If we are to keep this movement alive, instead of having it just another blip on what is popular in healthcare then our responsibility is to speak to the fact that working with people whose cultural values differ greatly from our own is a great challenge and will change us at every level. And the end result is negotiating an interaction that will allow for provision of excellent healthcare. I would love some feedback on this.

Rather than promoting the acquisition of specific knowledge or skills, Cooper's numerous posts indicate that she sees herself as part of a broader social movement dedicated to ending racism and achieving equal health care access for all.[10] For Cooper, the "business case" for cultural competence is less important than the ethical obligation to eliminate discrimination in health care. The "humane ethical virtues" of cultural competence are being encapsulated in modularized knowledge that, in Cooper's view, fails to deliver on the social justice mission of antiracism.

In response to this post, Bruce Daniels, a diversity consultant, suggested that expertise in cultural competency requires recognizing the limits of your knowledge. As he mounted a defense of standardized cultural competence training, Daniels drew out the fast-food metaphor by showing

---

10. Similar to CAHC practitioners who see themselves as part of a broad-based movement for social justice, some British homeopaths interviewed by Sarah Cant and Ursula Sharma see homeopathy as "a social movement [for a kind of health care] that should be made as accessible as possible." These homeopaths tended to oppose accreditation for homeopaths because it would lead to exclusivity in its search for "respectability" (1996, 584).

how even McDonald's has diversified its (standard) offerings. He nicely articulated the friction between biomedical expertise and the culturally specific, individualized expertise required by cultural competency:

> I think there is a place for "fast food cultural competence" as part of a spectrum or tool kit of cultural competence interventions that organizations and individuals choose from. . . . Fast food restaurants stand side by side with 5 star restaurants, in part because they serve different needs. When I was in New York as a recently diagnosed diabetic I got Asian and Caesar salads at McDonalds and they served my needs in a cost-effective way. Can we learn something here? I would recommend considering the concept of "cultural humility" coined by Melanie Tervalon and Jann Murray-Garcia to add to the discussion. Cultural humility means recognizing that we can't know everything about a culture, even one of our own. (I learn about being Black in this country every day! . . .) Cultural humility requires lifelong learning, self examination of our identities, biases and strengths, advocacy for both individual patients and populations facing discrimination, and a willingness to admit what we don't know. If we have the cultural humility to learn from a one hour video and provide some just in time education for that nurse caring for her Somali patient, we may help our patients and inspire our colleagues to engage in the lifelong learning that we love!

A diversity trainer himself, Daniels concluded that the imperative of standardized knowledge outweighs an individualized approach, as he specializes in providing cultural expertise for health care providers that enables them to more efficiently treat diverse patients (Anderson, Tang, and Blue 2007).[11]

In contrast, Jennifer Beck, a trainer who frequently promotes her book on cultural differences in health care on the list, joined Cooper in her lament of the quick training approach to cultural competency that many health care organizations and administrators want. Beck also pointed to administrators' acquiescence to industry and federal quality standards,

---

11. Bruce Daniels's use of the phrase "just in time education" sans scare quotes also invites comment. In late Fordist economies, just-in-time (JIT) production, as Deborah Leslie and David Butz (1998) have shown, shifts the burden of responding to fluctuating demand to line workers, whose hours may be extended or shrunk according to demand. Previously, managers would stock inventory in warehouses to satisfy demand. JIT production has been blamed for increased overtime hours (including unpaid hours), worker injury, and other hazards. Daniels's use of the term here to refer to education about Somali culture "for that nurse caring for her Somali patient" implies that cultural information and education, like products, can be disseminated on an as-needed basis and in a timely fashion such that the "customer" (the Somali patient) receives her "order" (quality, culturally appropriate health care) efficiently without wasting any extra time (money, information, or education) on extraneous principles such as fairness, respect, or equality.

yet she noted that compliance does not necessarily mean true engagement with the social change mission of CAHC. Therefore, unlike Daniels, Beck advocated organizational change, instead of admitting the usefulness of the "quick bite" approach. She wrote:

> I'm so glad there are so many of us of like minds! I've been researching, writing and teaching cultural and linguistic competency full time for the better part of 15 years and feel I've barely scratched the surface! I just love it when prospective clients want me to do (and I have been asked many times!) a how-to list for caring for patients from as many as 10 population groups and roll this out in an hour's presentation or write it for their web site! I've also had health care organizations order a copy of my book, telling me that JCAHO was visiting them the following week!

This discussion was recapped a couple of years later in response to a query from Richard, a poster whose job title was listed in his e-mail signature as "transformation agent" for a state mental health agency. Richard asked for suggestions for a "web-based rapid access tool for learning about or exploring more about a variety of cultures? I am currently looking for ways to utilize technology to make information available across our state." After several replies that included links for online education modules, the list received the following reply from a poster whose Web site identified him as professor of intercultural psychology at a European university:

> The postings on this topic aroused my curiosity and I had a look at two of the sites mentioned. . . . To my amazement I found myself back in the 1990s, when "cultural competence" was just a matter of finding the right stereotype to apply to your patient. With a few clicks of the mouse you would know everything about the person you were dealing with, just by looking up the properties of their "culture"! It has been a long, hard struggle to persuade people that matters are not as simple as that, and it kind of bothers me that in 2009 this approach is again being promoted as a solution—even as the solution—to the issue of diversity in health care. Let's just run through the objections again.
>
> 1. "Nationality" is not the same as "culture."
> 2. Cultures are neither homogeneous nor static. Within each cultural group there is great diversity, and cultures are in constant flux.
> 3. The fact that one can find statistically significant mean differences between national or cultural groups when they are administered simple questionnaires, says nothing about the

predictive value of these questionnaires. Why not? Because the variation within groups may be much greater than the variation between them (see point 2). Moreover, we know little about the relation between the way people answer questionnaires and the way they actually behave.

4. Almost by definition, migrants have been exposed to many influences beside[s] the culture(s) of their country of origin—one cannot assume that they will be typical of their country.

5. Last, and perhaps most important: people do not like being treated in stereotypical ways, simply as "a typical Filipino" or "a typical American"! Most people hate it!

Does this mean we should throw away the concept of "culture"? Absolutely not—we should simply recognise its complexity. The concept has helped people to realise that there are more ways of looking at the world besides their own, and that is a great step forward. But there is no "quick fix" for making health systems responsive to cultural diversity. Learning to communicate with someone who is different from you can never be achieved in a couple of mouse clicks: it is a matter of listening—which above all takes time—and being critical about one's own presuppositions.

I thought all this was boringly familiar by now, but even in the "diversity and health" community there seem to be some pretty big cultural differences. Does "web-based" always have to mean "simplistic and stereotypical"?

This response in turn earned replies from at least eight posters who repeated many of the points raised in the "fast-food" cultural competency thread presented previously, indicating that this online community of health care workers is still very much in the throes of defining both the limits and capacities of standardized cultural expertise.

Similarly, Gloria Zavella, a diversity coordinator with a state public health system, described the challenges of trying to achieve CAHC through organizational change. Echoing the language of the poster just quoted (though her post predated his by a couple of years), Zavella wrote, "There is no easy fix because it is an ongoing learning that never ends. This learning is associated with a curiosity about other cultures and a desire to understand and incorporate it in your daily work. For the organization, this means trans-organizational change at every level: the way we think, the way we work, the way we problem solve. My biggest challenge is getting hospital leaders and decision makers to understand this. It is not easy." In this comment, cultural expertise is linked with an enlightened subjectivity for health care providers as well as broader organizational change. While participants acknowledge the importance of establishing their expertise with the commonly accepted tools of the business of health care (such as outcome measures), they want to use these tools to rebuild the master's house from their liberal blueprint. Posters to the list grapple with the utility of applying instrumental rationality to achieve culturally appropriate health care. Technological reason dictates the need to emphasize the "business case" for culturally appropriate health care. *Making* CAHC technological itself—by developing standardized knowledge modules to disseminate cultural expertise, or by using the Internet to overcome limitations of time and space in its dissemination—may generate its own concerns, some of which were articulated in responses to a 2006 article by Arthur Kleinman and Peter Benson that was discussed at length on the list.[12] Among those defending Kleinman and Benson's critique, author Jennifer Beck disavowed a "technical" approach to cultural competence:

> Because I do offer a short summary and generalization of the common traditional health/illness beliefs of different cultures in my own book . . . I, too, have been accused of promoting stereotypes. I really try to avoid this. I have always advised caregivers not to merely assume that any individual patient will adhere to common beliefs attributed to those of their ethnicity, but to ask that patient questions which elicit his or her unique belief system. I agree [with Kleinman and Benson] that "cultural assumptions may hinder practical understanding," but feel background knowledge about the patient's presumed cultural group and language can be helpful to the caregiver in interpreting what the patient says in answer to such questions as, "What do you think has caused this illness? . . ." or any of the other questions in the Explanatory Models Approach. . . . [But] I don't think cultural competency is a technical skill that can be "mastered."

Despite elaborating here what has been called the "cultural content" approach to cultural competence ("background knowledge about the patient's cultural group and language"), Beck pointed to the limits of cultural expertise by suggesting that there is no mastery of cultural content because individual variation supersedes the possible gains from a technical approach. She continued, "Competency is the understanding that even then, after careful questioning, one cannot 'know' that individual completely and that continued ethnographic questioning is required throughout

---

12. In their paper "Anthropology in the Clinic: The Problem of Cultural Competency and How to Fix It" (2006), Arthur Kleinman and Peter Benson question the single-minded focus on "culture" seen in many cultural competency programs. Kleinman and Benson suggest that giving clinicians a laundry list of cultural traits they can use to type patients may in fact do more harm than good, inhibiting meaningful communication that would enable the clinician to understand the patient as an individual situated in a social world.

the entire treatment process." In the technological and social context of a list designed to build and foster the expertise of culture, Beck's argument *resists* the adequacy of cultural expertise and instead highlights the limits to knowing patients or cultures. Yet she rehabilitates the concept of competency by understanding it as the ability to perceive limits on knowledge, unlike the universalizing biomedical knowledge she critiques. She concluded with a different type of instrumental reasoning by offering the following political-economic analysis of health care: "What most desperately 'needs to be fixed' is a medical system that requires caregivers to see X number of patients in an hour and that fosters snap unilateral judgments by a caregiver who has not been given the time to take into consideration either the patient as an individual or his or her 'local world.'"

Others (e.g., Anderson, Tang, and Blue 2007) have elaborated on the political-economic critique with which Beck concluded her post. Joan Anderson and colleagues place the magnetic pull of standardized knowledge about culture in the context of overall health care restructuring, suggesting that "as a way of managing . . . heavy workloads in clinical settings, health care providers fall back on categories they believe will allow them to provide efficient care to patients and, at the same time, display cultural sensitivity" (2007, 304). A combination of economic and political forces have helped build the technologies of culturally appropriate health care explored here—technologies that are designed to achieve ethical goals yet which themselves come to function, Kleinman and Benson (2006) argue, in instrumental ways with their own unintended consequences.

Just as empowerment sits uneasily alongside employment programs as discussed in Chapter 3, list posters seek to balance exquisitely limited resources with ever-expanding knowledge requirements, including the dissemination of new forms of cultural knowledge. In doing so, list members must not only intervene in the debate between "standardization" and "individualization" that governs much health care practice and education; they must also take part in the dissemination of techniques that aim to transform the conditions of health care in order to bring to the center the concerns of marginalized groups. Cultural competence advocates straddle the divide between the standardization of knowledge commonly seen in continuing medical education courses and "individualization," the time-consuming process of learning about a patient in a tailored approach.[13] Efficiency, accountability, and QI, as "techniques of instrumental reason," have also been used to rationalize changes aimed at making health care more culturally appropriate. In contrast to moral philosophers who view technological reason as standing apart from or in opposition to ethics,

---

13. See also Cheryl Mattingly's description of individualized treatment in contrast with "standardized, measureable treatment goals that stay within clear disciplinary boundaries" (1998, 279).

Stephen Collier and Andrew Lakoff, in their introduction to the collection *Global Assemblages*, touch on the diverse ways in which technological reason has become intertwined with questions of values. "As Max Weber and others have argued, the techniques of instrumental reason are of increasingly broad ethical significance across the life worlds. The extension of such techniques can be understood as constantly provoking new 'ethical' questions as concrete forms of technological reason enter into dynamic, productive, and often problematic relations with values" (Collier and Lakoff 2005, 28). In fact, forms of technological reason such as QI produce broader effects as well, changing our understandings of what it is to be both human and ethical. Collier and Lakoff continue, "Technological reason is continually involved in constituting 'human nature' and diverse ethical subjects" (2005, 28). Similarly, cultural competence training works to constitute human nature as "cultural" while promoting new forms of expertise such as "cultural competence." The process through which mapping and knowing communities is also about governing them, as discussed in Chapter 2, is reflected in the instrumentalization of "culture" as it is enacted in technologies of culturally appropriate health care.

Technological reason dictates the terms in which actors (both culturally competent doctors and culturally identified patients) act, as well as the terms in which cultural competence trainings can be considered effective. List members often post requests for "tools" or "instruments" that would allow them to demonstrate the effectiveness of the expensive cultural competence trainings that they would like to purchase for health care providers in their organizations. For example, a language services manager at a midwestern hospital wrote, "I am working on a budget report to obtain more full-time positions for our department, and in the report I would like to include a few facts or at least reference to any study that shows the positive effect (i.e., patient satisfaction, better health outcome, lower expenditure over the long term, etc.) of providing language services. . . . I am looking for something external to put in to give the report extra oomph. Thanks in advance!" Another participant observed, "One of the things we have discovered is that a lot of the previous work is 'global' and somewhat general and/or academic. While that foundation is good, applying the work to the context of compliance, quality patient care, etc. has helped tremendously. This can appear to be basic, but it really helps leadership and staff/providers start to clearly grasp what is being done, and why it is important. The underlying mission, vision, and value of culturally competent care will grow in value and strength and really 'win a hearing.'"

Ideally, technologies of culturally appropriate health care are designed to produce legible *outcomes* such as increased patient safety, improved patient satisfaction, and so on, though in practice this data is scarce. As a result, many CC promoters fall back on ethical justifications rather than effectiveness claims for CC training and CAHC. Through its assignation to QI departments in health care organizations, CAHC becomes folded in with issues such as treatment compliance, quality improvement, or patient safety. List members function as cultural brokers on the border between two worlds—the "soft" worlds of medical anthropology, cultural relativism, human rights, and patient-centered care, and the "hard" worlds of positivism, empiricism, universalizing biomedical expertise, and the unavoidable demands for efficiency. Between these, Culture and Health list members and those seeking to insert cultural expertise into the knowledge economies of health care are trying to demonstrate to administrators why cultural competence programs are important.

Discussing the increasing encroachment of economic rationalities into social and governmental domains that previously were governed by other ethical or political norms such as equity or justice, Rose observes, "The emphasis on defined and measurable goals and targets in the work that professionals do with their clients is an element within a much wider reconfiguration of methods for the government of specialist activities" (1999, 154). For example, some list members argue that final justification for cultural expertise can be provided only by quantified evidence of effectiveness. A Swiss medical anthropologist wrote, "We are all convinced that what we do is important, but there isn't nearly enough direct evidence out there to support our position, so we should be investing more efforts in this important but difficult area of research, otherwise we risk being written off as simply doing what is 'politically correct.'" In contrast, another member questioned the existence of outcomes research for health communication skills more generally:

> However, not much outcomes research has been done on *any* well-specified communications or interactional skills in medicine. And, for that matter, little research has been done that demonstrates specific types or levels of clinician knowledge and patient outcomes. It is a whole lot harder to design and carry out such research than it is to correlate the number of specific surgical procedures performed with patient outcomes, but maybe someone should try.[14]

Hinting at ambivalence toward cultural expertise and the technologies they develop, list members both seek new technologies to demonstrate the effectiveness of their knowledge and resist the widespread use of those technologies, in part because of their essentializing and reductionistic tendencies

---

14. Indeed, the evidence based medicine (EBM) movement would suggest that little of what is currently established medical practice has actually been "proven effective." For reviews of some of the controversies associated with the effort to institute EBM in the United States, see Feinstein and Horwitz 1997, Denny 1999, and Lambert 2006. See also Rock 2005 and Hay et al. 2008 for ethnographic contributions to this literature.

(sometimes even using those very terms of critique). These responses do nothing to add value to cultural competency programs, however, and thus are shared only in a "like minds" context such as this list. More broadly, cultural competence promoters do their part to instrumentalize cultural competence as they strive to produce justifications for cultural expertise that articulate with the instrumental logical of health care (QI, patient safety, cost-effectiveness, health outcomes).

Conclusion

These new forms of expertise are part of what Nikolas Rose (1998) terms the "relocation" of the state as nonstate and quasi-state organizations such as the Joint Commission now uphold (formerly) state responsibilities for ensuring equality, access, and public health. The trainings, orientations, assessments, and policies that make up culturally appropriate health care function, in Rose's words, as a *"technique for the disciplining of human difference*: individualizing humans through classifying them, calibrating their capacities and conducts . . . managing and utilizing their individuality and variability" (Rose 1998, 19). The political problems of inequitable access to health care, and care that discriminates against the poor and people of color, are being reconstructed as technical barriers to quality health care that are renamed "cultural difference." CAHC builds on early "culture studies" approaches to manage broader social and political contestation over goods and services, but it should not be understood as a monolithic knowledge formation. Constituted through contestation among participants over ethics, aims, and strategies, CAHC is simultaneously stabilized by forces such as the CLAS regulations and the Joint Commission's revisions to its annual survey of health care organizations. The state (for example, the U.S. Office of Minority Health) hopes to resolve contestation around cultural difference in the clinic by issuing regulations mandating liberal forms of accommodation and equal access.[15] Making cultural difference a problem of regulated social interaction, technologies of CAHC address cultural differences in clinical settings through a variety of measures, such as consent forms in multiple languages and the location of health services in certain neighborhoods. Among such reforms, the most critical, and thus my focus here, are the education of health care providers on culture and health and the reorganization of health care systems to accommodate the needs of patients from diverse backgrounds. An ethico-

---

15. For example, Title VI of the Civil Rights Act mandates that health care providers (and all recipients of federal funding) provide interpretation services to those who are not proficient in English, though no federal funding is provided to support those interpreters. On the basis of this statute, the CLAS regulations mandate language access for health care providers, while the other eleven items in the regulations are "guidelines" rather than mandates.

political problem of justice and equality is sorted out through procedures designed to produce equal outcomes if not identical practices. Technologies of CAHC are amalgamated into broader processes of governmental reflexivity (Rose 1999, 7), whose terms are set by neoliberal transformations in governing that emphasize the paradoxical values of efficiency, standardization, and flexibility. Through the CLAS mandates, the state shifts responsibility for addressing problems of access to health care related to cultural and language differences to health care providers with neither reimbursement nor enforcement mechanisms. In addition to delegating responsibility for ensuring equality to health care providers, these policies may deflect attention from broader structural influences on health disparities.

At the end of the roundtable on evaluating CC trainings discussed earlier, Margaret encouraged the audience to "not to get stuck on the individual level" when thinking about how to define cultural competence. "I suggest to you," she continued, "that it's very difficult to be a culturally competent physician [or] nurse in an organization that does not support it with policies, procedures, and resources. We really need to look at training as an aspect, and not the primary aspect, for helping people to move along the continuum of cultural competence." Margaret emphasized organizational change as the most important factor in reducing disparities in quality of care. While cultural competence advocates see themselves at the forefront of an antiracist movement that seeks to extend this awareness to others, they simultaneously acknowledge their failure to address the structural factors that determine the health disparities that opened this movement. Advocacy groups mobilizing for remedies to racial and ethnic health disparities point to a wide range of factors, including discrimination in health care settings and social determinants such as poverty, segregation, access to care, and health insurance as sources of health disparities (Chapman and Berggren 2005). Another speaker observed that most "awareness tools" focus on being comfortable with and knowledgeable about different cultural groups, which she worried "might take attention away from what we really need to do to address the underlying factors."[16] The CHA program discussed in Chapters 2 and 3 is another example of programs developed at an organizational level to increase health care access.

While, as Paul Rabinow notes, "it is generally recognized within anthropology that the 'culture' concept raises more questions than it solves" (2005, 46), in medicine and public health the culture concept is flourishing under federal regulations that require health care organizations to offer

---

16. Tomas Matza makes an analogous argument about "political technologies like [discourses of] self-esteem" in mediating social conflict in contemporary Russia. Matza observes that these discourses become "paradoxically antipolitical technologies because discontent is obscured by the endeavor of affective engagement, and the zone for political work remains at the level of the self" (2009, 513).

care that is "culturally and linguistically appropriate" (Geary 2007). The Culture and Health list and the Internet both provide opportunities for cultural experts to build and disseminate their expertise, reconstructing and often reifying the concept of cultural difference among populations in the process. Shaped by demands for efficiency and replicability, technologies of culturally appropriate health care bring unintended consequences that include the reification of ethnic categories. Cultural competence education faces the challenge of fitting the project of cultural relativism into standardized forms of knowledge. And constructing approaching cultural difference in the clinic as a technical problem continues to obscure structural causes of health disparities while it creates new and often reductive understandings of the meaning of difference.

II

Technologies of Prevention and Boundaries of Citizenship

Drug Use, Research, and Public Health

erms such as *community*, *culture*, and *difference* become disaggregated into collections of practices and beliefs as we examine their multiple meanings in community health. Subject positions for health care workers are shaped by diverse forces, including the political economy of health care, visions of community mobilization, and concepts of community and difference. The CHA program designers described in Part I imagined their community in ethnic terms; community was a relational vision in which people bound together by a shared ethnic identity choose a common course of action. However, as explored further in Part II, the issue of identity is almost immediately problematized by making claims "on behalf of" any putatively bounded group. Any unity asserted for political purposes is capable of being fractured from within by those who assert difference within the unity or by others who seek to draw lines of exclusion against those who fail to meet criteria of community membership through their dependence on the state or on illicit drugs.

The following two chapters explore another aspect of Thornton, that populated by those most at risk for HIV infection. To the preceding analysis of health care providers' efforts to manage cultural difference in the clinic, the ethnographic research presented in Part II adds detailed exploration of the social production of marginalized populations and the role of community health knowledge and practice in facilitating that process. Chapter 5 examines the ways in which risk categories articulate populations and how members of these populations act on risk information in unanticipated ways. While political economists such as Merrill Singer (2004) show how drug users are under-served and marginalized by the state, governmentality theorists analyze how states are charged with promoting the health of those populations produced by risk analyses (Miller 2001a). Yet, as described in Chapter 6, drug users are problematically "us" and "not-us," at times part of the body politic whose health is protected by the state, at times ejected therefrom as state constructions of drug use and addiction oscillate between disease and criminality.

The vexed intersection of substance abuse and HIV is a key site where "governmentality" hits the ground (Mugford 1993; Valverde 1998). How do HIV prevention programs work to manage the capacities and habits of drug users? In what ways can programs such as syringe exchange be understood as grassroots solutions to the epidemic? Critical analyses of social responses to drug use and addiction open a "new perspective on . . . the relationship between state and society, the key rationales and tools of government, and the concrete sites and technologies employed in the for-mation and governance of social subjects" (Fischer et al. 2004, 358). In the chapters that follow, I explore the circulation of harm reduction discourse through federally funded drug research to uncover the ways in which researchers and drug users alike are constructed in the research encounter (Chapter 5). Applied social research, completed to identify new and better ways to prevent HIV infections among those most at risk, contributes to the construction of new concepts of risk that ramify in unexpected ways. A discourse of empowerment associated with harm reduction empha-sizes individual responsibility for managing risks associated with drug use (Erickson et al. 1997; Miller 2001a). Harm reduction interventions such as syringe exchange programs, the focus of Chapter 6, are simultaneously a population-based risk management approach (in seeking to increase the availability of sterile syringes and thus prevent HIV infections among injection drug users) and an individualized one, relying on users to regu-larly attend the exchange for syringes and to inject with a sterile syringe every time. Syringe exchange programs enact their accountability to their funders and the public as they keep strict track of the syringes they put into circulation. They enforce similar regimes of accountability for drug users, requiring them to retain their used syringes to exchange for new ones. At the same time, harm reduction programs provide an alternative ethics of drug use that seeks to demonstrate respect for those who use drugs and modify society in order to make drug use less harmful. The uneasy balance between these two interpretations of harm reduction colors local debates over HIV prevention programs as well as their implementation.

Thornton's residents, like people elsewhere (Abel 2005; Bluthenthal 1998; Egelko 2009; Broadhead, van Hulst, and Heckathorn 1999), have struggled with decisions about the best way to respond to drug use, alter-nately participating in and contesting representations of addiction as either illness or crime. In Thornton, as elsewhere, public beliefs and expectations about HIV prevention vary enormously regarding the proper role of government in protecting and promoting public health and safety. As in community health and policy responses to the "problem" of cultural difference in the clinic, HIV prevention measures are a site of contestation where participants struggle over the meanings of identity, belonging, citizenship, and entitlement.

Especially in domains involving HIV/AIDS, health care and research, as practices of governance, actively construct subject-positions for individuals through the transmission of information about risk (Robertson 2001) that implies certain obligations for actions to protect the self and others (Brownlie and Howson 2006; Koch and Svendsen 2005). Like the community health programs outlined in Part I, HIV prevention programs function as a technique of governing at the same time that they serve the interests of disenfranchised groups. Chapter 6 traces local struggles over the implementation of HIV prevention programs for injection drug users, outlining the ways in which responses to HIV are driven by the same liberal mandate to expand access to care and prevention, while facing unique complications posed by the criminal justice interpretation of drug use.

While the prevailing AIDS prevention ideology is that "anyone can get AIDS," certain populations are both perceived as and in fact more at risk for AIDS and HIV. In Massachusetts, the most commonly reported mode of exposure to HIV among all women living with HIV/AIDS is injection drug use. Most women living with AIDS are black (42 percent, up from 36 percent of women with AIDS in 2001) and Hispanic (28 percent) (MDPH 2010, 2001). In Thornton in 2001, significantly more people have been infected with HIV through injection drug use compared to both the state and the United States as a whole (44 percent of people living with AIDS in Thornton were infected through injection drug use, versus 31 percent in Massachusetts and 20 percent nationwide). AIDS in Thornton continues to be much more prevalent among people of color than in the rest of the state, with more than twice the percentage of people with AIDS who are Hispanic. So while the Puerto Rican program coordinator at a nearby SEP agency commented to me in an in-depth interview, "It can affect [Fairfield, an affluent white suburb of Thornton]. It can affect [Claremont, another suburb]. It can affect anyone," Chris Collins, the white program director, responded.

It *can*, but it doesn't seem to. I mean, when I look at the question of how [AIDS] affects work and at home, . . . you know, I see HIV in the community as just another one of those divisive issues that—that really separates, white middle-class, upper-middle-class people from communities of color. You know . . . , it's really clear to me that the majority of the decision makers in [Thornton] think,

"Well, that's . . . the Puerto Ricans' problem, you know, and they're—they're a guest in our city. They're *unwelcome* guests here." You know.

The sociopolitical and economic context of AIDS risk in Thornton is shaped by shrinking public resources for social programs. HIV infection is intensified in Thornton's vulnerable populations by the process of deindustrialization beginning in the 1970s at the tail end of waves of northern immigration of southern African Americans and Puerto Ricans (Bourgois 1995); declining housing stock and homeownership among African American and Hispanic inner-city residents following urban renewal programs of the 1950s and 1960s (Fullilove 2001); underfunded public schools; and lack of access to sterile syringes over the counter or from syringe exchange programs (Neaigus et al. 2008). The combination of these factors makes up what Allen Feldman (2001) calls *conditions of advanced marginalization*.

Several community-based organizations in Thornton serve the populations at increased risk for HIV, including the partner organizations in the CHA program described previously (Helping the Black Family, TCHC, El Pueblo, the Brighton Square drop-in center). During my fieldwork, their most common funding source for HIV prevention programs serving drug users was the Massachusetts Department of Public Health, which experienced major funding cuts beginning in 2001. Outreach workers in Thornton were a tight-knit group, though employed by different agencies. All told similar stories about the challenges of trying to do HIV prevention work with people who were actively using drugs, yet none were able to locate enough drug treatment programs for those clients who expressed the desire to stop or at least reduce their drug use.

In addition to structural factors that put marginalized groups at increased risk for addiction and limit their access to drug treatment programs, stigma plays an important role in the social construction of drug users. Injection drug users (IDUs) are stigmatized as dependent on drugs, the state, or both (Campbell 2000; Glick Schiller, Crystal, and Lewellen 1994; Reinarman and Levine 1997; Valverde 1998). A news article from the South Florida *Sun-Sentinel*, describing attendees of a syringe exchange program in Puerto Rico, provides a vivid image that could serve as an archetype of the stigmatized IDU: "They arrive gaunt and red-eyed, some wobbling on rusty bicycles, others casting a wary eye as they walk quickly onto the dusty courtyards of this city's housing projects. Most carry their needles in bunches of twos and threes, but others bring dozens in bags and small boxes" (Collie 2001, 1A). Raising the specter of the drug-addicted mother that haunts many outcries against drug users (Campbell 2000), the lead paragraph of this front-page article concludes, "One woman carries 47 [used syringes] in a disposable-diaper box" (Collie 2001, 1A).

Such descriptions of "gaunt" drug users who are unable to properly move around ("wobbling on rusty bicycles") signify governing mentalities of drug use that highlight the failure of IDUs to care for themselves. While others have explored the racialized stigmatization of people of color as drug users and addicts (especially injection drug users [Singer 1999] and crack cocaine users [Fullilove, Lown, and Fullilove 1992]), in my view it is the social construction of drug users as *dependent* in their (risk of) addiction that is the root of their stigmatization (Valverde 1998)—a stigma that is differentially elaborated in particular, racialized ways for different groups.

Part II draws on findings from two related NIH-supported studies completed between 2001 and 2005. The Syringe Access study included epidemiological surveys with 989 injection drug users in three New England cities (Thornton, Massachusetts; Hartford, Connecticut; and New Haven, Connecticut), plus a variety of ethnographic research methods.[1] The Community Attitudes study focused on local struggles over state-sponsored syringe exchange to prevent HIV infection among injection drug users and involved a door-to-door survey of residents of five Thornton neighborhoods, participant-observation research in public meetings and hearings where syringe exchange was debated, and in-depth interviews with syringe exchange staff members in nearby cities in Massachusetts and Connecticut.[2]

1. The study was funded by the National Institute on Drug Abuse (R01 DA12569, Merrill Singer, Principal Investigator).
2. The study was funded by the National Institute on Drug Abuse (R03 DA16532, Susan Shaw, Principal Investigator).

5

"I Always Use Bleach"

The Production and Circulation of
Risk and Norms in Drug Research

"I always use bleach—I never share my needles." An injection drug user (IDU) speaking to a researcher knows this is the appropriate thing to say when she is asked, "Do you [how often do you, why do you] share your needles?" In ethnographic research I conducted on HIV risk among people who inject drugs in Thornton, participants repeated variations on these themes while I observed them getting high and interviewed them about their "risk practices." They sometimes would repeat these mantras as they failed to use bleach or even used their partner's needle before my eyes. This disjunction between narrative and behavior led me to ask: How do IDUs come to know what they *should* say in response to our interview questions? How were these norms created by the harm reduction movement and public health educators? And finally, what is the role of researchers in the creation, dissemination, and recognition of harm reduction norms?

Following cultural policy analyses by Nancy Campbell (2000) and others (Shore and Wright 1997; Hyatt 2001), this chapter offers an inquiry into the role of research in constructing populations, mobilizing risk, and disseminating norms aimed at the self-government of drug users. I consider the possible unintended consequences of researchers' intense focus on the risk behaviors that increase the chances of HIV transmission. By isolating behavioral factors that increase "risk" for HIV, I argue, drug researchers construct discrete new populations that did not exist before the research in the same way as they did subsequent to it. The "injection drug user"—a frequent subject of many studies—is one example of such categorizing. The specification of populations such as "injection drug users" functions as a technique of governing when it leads to new knowledge or programs (e.g., the "supervised injection sites" described by Benedikt Fischer and colleagues in a special issue of *International Journal of Drug Policy* [2004]). My experience as ethnographer on the multi-investigator Syringe Access study[1] brought home to me the extent to which participants associate drug researchers with certain behavioral norms ("clean your works [injection paraphernalia] with bleach," "don't share needles") that are clearly *morally valued* (Fischer et al. 2004) and socially rewarded. Further, ethnographically informed representations of risk shape users' understandings of what kinds of objects and practices represent danger, in sometimes unexpected ways. I conclude by considering the implications of relying exclusively on behavior-based risk categories to describe the HIV epidemic. My concern is that drug researchers lean toward becoming technocrats when research relies on behavior-based risk categories to the exclusion of other social and structural factors, omitting the potential for organizing in response to health threats (see, for example, Chapter 6) that may draw on facets of identity obscured in populations designated through behavior alone.

For years, anthropologists and others have called for greater understanding and analysis of the social context of HIV risk (Singer et al. 1992; Singer 1993). We argue that appropriate interventions cannot be developed unless and until we understand the fullness and complexity of the lives of those at highest risk for HIV. Ethnographic work reveals the interrelationships between poverty, homelessness, racism, and other forms of structural violence as they shape HIV risk for diverse populations (Singer 1994a, 1999). While these studies can be and are used to make interventions more appropriate for the real circumstances faced by people at risk for and living with HIV, we must also consider the implications of our contributions to rendering HIV risk knowable, identifiable, and understandable. I am interested in the ways in which drug users have come to see researchers as embodying harm reduction, and, more specifically, HIV prevention norms, and how this has come to supersede traditional perceptions of researchers and policy makers as embodying the norm of abstinence.

---

1. This multisite study funded by the National Institute on Drug Abuse (R01 DA12569, Merrill Singer, Principal Investigator) examined the micro- and macro-level factors that shape HIV risk for IDUs in three northeastern cities (Thornton, Massachusetts, and two sites in Connecticut). A team of researchers from the Hispanic Health Council, Yale University, and the University of Massachusetts used epidemiological, qualitative, and bioassay methods to identify and compare factors in HIV and hepatitis C risk at the individual, neighborhood, and city levels. In addition to quantitative surveys, ethnographers at each site completed several types of "activities" including in-depth interviews (in which we collected life and drug use histories); syringe acquisition interviews; and drug use observations.

On Epidemiology, Ethnography, and Risk

Funded in large part by a government apparatus bent on extracting "data" from ethnographic representations of "risky practices" for the sake of better governing the public health, drug ethnographers, like the outreach workers profiled in Part I, have historically helped uncover hidden behaviors and populations, thus making them available for intervention. Drug ethnographers collect data in the form of ethnographic stories, observations, and quantitative surveys about what users actually do when they use drugs (e.g., Broadhead and Fox 1990; Clatts 1995). The appearance of HIV/AIDS and the epidemiological association between HIV transmission and needle sharing drove the expansion of both the epidemiological and ethnographic enterprises funded by federal agencies such as the National Institute on Drug Abuse (NIDA) in the mid- to late 1980s (Campbell and Shaw 2008; Herdt and Lindenbaum 1992; Roe 2005). Epidemiologists set out a typology of risk group categories that proved problematic for drug ethnographers but also tipped the policy balance away from viewing drug use through a criminological lens and toward viewing it as a public health problem. Gradually, NIDA became more open to supporting ethnographic research on drug use, and public health was a frequent justification for conducting ethnographic work with so-called hidden populations.

Specifying just what members of "hidden populations," previously inaccessible to large-scale data collection efforts, *did* while using drugs (or having sex) gradually led to the production of increasingly fine-grained differentiations between "risk groups" or drug subcultures (Campbell and Shaw 2008). Governing the health of a population through the cataloging of discrete populations and then regulating their behaviors is accomplished in part through the production and circulation of information about risk. Risk has become a key governing mentality of both ethnographic and epidemiological approaches to the HIV epidemic, with wide-ranging effects that have reached both harm reduction workers and policy makers.[2] Robert Castel (1991) and others (e.g., Petersen 1997; Wynne 2001; Lash, Szerszynski, and Wynne 1996) have described the production of risk through regimes of power/knowledge. The risk society they describe has created a structure of feeling that includes a climate of anxiety in which "everybody is compelled to be on guard" (Jones 2004, 368). Drug users must endeavor to protect themselves and others from HIV infection, while

---

2. Nancy Campbell defines governing mentalities as "the frames in which truth claims make sense. The assumptions and images that compose the governing mentalities [of drug discourses] also structure the apparatus of knowledge production" (2000, 34). I draw on the concept of governing mentalities here to introduce multiplicity into the concept of governmentality, and to indicate the simultaneous coexistence of regulatory regimes working along multiple dimensions to constitute highly differentiated populations for the sake of managing risk.

members of the "general population" fear IDUs because of their addiction as well as place- and race-based stigma (Wacquant 1993). The deployment of risk discourse in public health is ineluctably about governance (Castel 1991; Roe 2005); rather than looking only at what is forbidden by risk management, we must consider what risk *enables*: the production of risk allows certain actors to *do* things that they could not otherwise accomplish, such as the institutionalization of "safe injection sites" (Small 2007) or prescription heroin. At the other end of the punitive spectrum, criminal transmission laws allow people with HIV infection to be imprisoned for spitting or for having unprotected sex (Altman 2008). As the assumptions of epidemiology became governing mentalities with the development of the AIDS epidemic, and as the focus of epidemiological research shifted from identity to behavior, populations were designated on the basis of "behavior" while the social, cultural, and structural forces that shape behavior receded from view (Lindenbaum 1992).

Ethnographic researchers also produced new behavioral categories to combat the stigma associated with the popularly and epidemiologically constituted notion of the first "risk groups" identified for HIV—IDUs and gay men. Anthropological critiques of the constitution of risk on the basis of identity argued that these stigmatized categories obscured more than they revealed (e.g., Clatts 1995). Behavioral risk categories were advanced at the beginning of the HIV/AIDS epidemic as benign alternatives to pejorative terms for drug users such as *junkie* or *addict* (Glick Schiller, Crystal, and Lewellen 1994). In the late 1980s and early 1990s, AIDS educators drilled into our heads, "It's not who you are, it's what you *do*" (Clatts 1995; see also Geary 2007). *Injection drug user* defined a population on the basis of activities understood to be "risky" for HIV infection. Millions of state and federal dollars have been spent researching, serving, and governing the population—IDUs—thus defined.

Anthropologists and others were presented with classificatory dilemmas borne of the limitations of the behavior-based risk categories that eventually supplanted stigmatizing identity-based risk groups. The epidemiological assumption that "subcultural" norms cause individuals to engage in risky behavior has been much criticized (e.g., Kane and Mason 1992; Farmer 1992), but fewer authors have addressed the limitations and exclusions of behavior-based risk categories. Epidemiological research that designates populations on the basis of behavior pins responsibility for health risks on individuals when it turns the analytic lens away from contributing social and structural factors (Petersen 1997; Nichter 2003; Moore and Fraser 2006).

Anthropological and epidemiological research on drug use and HIV risk has contributed to the construction of a range of new categories constituted in this effort to protect and promote the public health. Ian Hacking (1986) proposes the idea of *dynamic nominalism* to describe the effects of categories on subjective consciousness or identity formation. He writes, "The claim of dynamic nominalism is . . . that a kind of person came into being at the same time as the kind itself was being invented" (1986, 228). In other words, "counting [populations] is no mere report of developments. It elaborately, often philanthropically, creates new ways for people to be. People spontaneously come to fit their categories" (223). Research has been a central discourse through which the construction of behavioral risk categories has metamorphosed into a subject-position (IDU) that is filled by an individual whose other layers of identity may be altered or even erased as he or she is enlisted in the public health project of HIV prevention.[3] Social movements and public health bureaucracies alike participate in the governance of populations as epidemiological constructions of risk are transformed into behavioral guidelines delivered through outreach and community-based interventions. Ethnographers played a key role in documenting and evaluating these interventions (Singer 2002), and gradually came to embody changing social norms in the communities they studied. Ethnographers are now understood to play an important role in anatomizing risky practices associated with patterns of needle use, but their role in the circulation of harm reduction narratives is less well recognized.

Hidden Histories of Harm Reduction

Harm reduction is a pragmatic social movement aimed at changing the personal practices of drug users through "modest interventions" designed to reduce negative health and social effects of drug use. Because harm reduction emerged simultaneously from several communities of practice beginning in the 1970s, there are multiple origin stories for harm reduction beliefs and practices (e.g., Erickson et al. 1997; O'Hare et al. 1992; Roe 2005). Cultivated and disseminated through research as well as direct-service and

---

3. Ironically, as behavior-based designations such as *IDU* erase the social and contextual information that *may* have been conveyed in, for example, the phrase "a forty-five-year-old Latino male," public health researchers are put in the somewhat awkward position of having to seek empirical evidence of the effects of structural factors concealed by the term *IDU*. In a related response, some readers express concern about my use of ethnic identifiers (white, African American, Latino) in descriptions of participants. These concerns typically come up around descriptions that have to do with drug use, but seldom elsewhere. I use such descriptors because, as I try to show in Part II, it is significant that low-income ethnic minorities are more likely than white middle-class participants both to take part in publicly funded drug research and to become infected with HIV as a result of their drug use. Without doubt, white, middle-class people in Thornton's suburbs use illicit drugs at rates similar to those of other groups, but they are less likely to be motivated by cash incentives to reveal their personal information to a stranger. I interviewed no middle-class drug users during the Syringe Access study (at least, none who disclosed themselves to me as such). If middle class, they may have more resources to conceal their drug use, resources that also help protect them from HIV infection and from the public health surveillance measures that accompany it.

advocacy organizations, harm reduction shapes users' self-definitions, conduct toward others, and control over things (drugs, blood, syringes, cotton). Harm reduction discourse serves as an alternative ethics to the ethics of both criminal justice and the medical discourse underlying public health approaches.[4] Harm reduction practices designed to prevent the transmission of HIV, such as bleaching used syringes before reuse, are shaped by epidemiological representations of HIV risk and transmission. However, harm reduction is also a critical discourse built on a humanistic view of drug users that preserves their intrinsic value and moral worth despite their engagement in illegal behaviors and the compulsions at work in addiction (Roe 2005). At the same time, harm reduction practices are used to navigate a neoliberal political rationality that relocates responsibility for health to individuals without addressing structural constraints or the cultural geography and social economy of drug markets (Moore and Fraser 2006). This chapter provides an ethnographic account of the travels of harm reduction discourse through federally funded drug ethnography and in everyday talk between drug users and researchers.

Harm reduction was simultaneously constructed through grassroots mobilization, outreach, and public health research (Riley and O'Hare 2000; Roe 2005). In the wake of the AIDS epidemic, many harm reduction interventions focus on reducing the risk of HIV transmission through contaminated injection equipment, a practice that runs afoul of the criminalization of drug use and drug paraphernalia such as syringes. Alternately repressed and promoted, harm reduction became a normative set of practices in public health arenas that have now expanded far beyond drug use and the attempt to contain HIV transmission (Nichter 2003). The governing mentalities of harm reduction thus reposition drug use as an ethical practice, making possible the idea that drug use should, for example, take place in a "safe space."[5]

Harm reduction further troubles the cultural fiction of an "abstinence-based" society with a consistent and effective drug policy. A vernacular uptake of an unofficial, "underground" discourse of harm reduction accompanied the circulation of official conceptualizations of illicit drug use or addiction, risk, and harm in public space (Feldman 2001). Despite its uncertain and even underground status, harm reduction discourse has circulated throughout drug treatment and HIV prevention programs and services. This discourse has become an alternative governing mentality and a set of normative practices that drug users know they should adopt

---

4. Historian Nancy Campbell sketches "the two seemingly oppositional frames that structure U.S. drug policy: 'crime' and 'disease'" in her book *Using Women*, on representations of women drug users in public debates and the media (2000, 45). See also Small 2007.

5. Benedikt Fischer and colleagues (2004) describe the political and ethical stance toward Australian drug users revealed by drug policies that include safe injection rooms and syringe distribution; see also Small 2007.

or, at the very least, report in epidemiological surveys conducted by social science researchers (Singer et al. 1992).

Harm Reduction Norms and Ethics

The strength of the injunctions established by harm reduction—*clean your works; don't share syringes*—was apparent during the Syringe Access study. One muggy summer day when Dwayne Rogers, the outreach worker we met in the Introduction, and the Thornton site investigator were collecting discarded syringes in an out-of-the-way park, they encountered a Latino couple who appeared to have just gotten high in the woods at the edge of the park. Although Rogers assured the couple that his colleague was a teacher engaged in research, not law enforcement, the researcher's photographs of discarded syringes nevertheless provoked enough discomfort that the woman blurted out, "We always use bleach!" Her assertion worked to constitute her as an ethical subject who understands the risks to which she is subject and who practices harm reduction techniques. Ritual invocations such as this have multiple aims, including shielding a user from further "intervention" and establishing ethical harmony between participant and researcher by demonstrating compliance with assumed behavioral norms for safety. Instead of accepting such statements as the endpoint of the investigation—as if HIV prevention were ensured—I use the answers that signal "we're done" as starting places for an epistemological inquiry about how those who study risk also embody norms.

"We always use bleach" and "I never share needles" are learned responses that invoke shared social and cultural norms of harm reduction that may be pronounced for more than one purpose. Ana Ning (2005), for example, explores the strategic acts of complicity that methadone clients engaged in as they worked to position themselves as ethical users in recovery:[6]

> Individual actions are not always what they appear to be. In the ensuing ethnographic examples both clients and staff are complicit with the discourses that they critique, meaning that they are both caught up in the complex workings of power, whereby neither is exclusively dominant or exclusively resistant to domination. After all, both are constituted by, and set within a social and political framework that may be either enabling or constraining their lives. (351)

---

6. Methadone is often prescribed as a substitute for people addicted to opiates (see Bourgois 2000). This usually involves daily attendance at a methadone clinic for a dose as well as occasional visits with a counselor who tracks a client's drug use practices and offers therapeutic support.

Ning interprets complicitous acts as creating an appearance of conformity while subverting dominant decision makers and converting treatment goals to better meet the needs of the marginalized. She, too, observed claims that diverged from actual practices, citing harm reduction as a contradictory discursive site: "When clients articulate the discourse of harm reduction, one could think that this discourse has been inculcated in them and that they have internalized it, with the result that they are in agreement with the ends of the treatment program. However, clients may appropriate these discourses to serve their own ends" (2005, 356). These aims including establishing the speaker as an ethical subject and a capable participant in state-sponsored drug ethnography.[7] Building on Nancy Campbell's work on the constitution of drug users as objects and subjects of knowledge (1995, 2000), I began an inquiry into the role of drug research in constructing populations, mobilizing risk, and performing harm reduction norms aimed at getting drugs users to adopt "protective" features of self-government.

Constituting Norms through Research

State-funded substance abuse researchers play both instrumental and expressive roles in the governance of drug use. Like all researchers, drug ethnographers shape the findings we collect, which affects the knowledge we create and the uses to which the data we produce are put. The governing mentalities of research also produce researchers who ask only certain kinds of questions and not others—for example, "How many times in the past thirty days have you shared syringes?" but not, "What is it like when you try to look for housing?" The perception that all the ethnographer looks for is an assurance that the subject is enacting harm reduction principles in daily practice has become a barrier to discerning actual practices as well as the broader structural constraints that shape them. Subjects anticipate questions and offer responses that suggest they approach the research relationship as one of quid pro quo (see Gupta and Sharma 2006, 289–290). The following exchange with Dave Wood, the user we met in the Introduction, drove that point home for me:

> Susan: So when you're using with other people, just socially—
> Dave: Do we share needles? No.
> Susan: [*Laughs.*]
> Dave: Go ahead. I'm sorry.
> Susan: Are you anticipating my questions?
> Dave: Listen, I don't play that.

---

7. For instance, I had participants volunteer to assist me in my research, bringing in printouts of Web pages they thought I might find useful, or offering to collect additional interviews for me.

By responding, "I don't play that," this career injector was not trying to cut off the conversation about risk so much as to establish that he was an ethical person who did not share needles (in a rhetorical move similar to that at the opening, where he tries to distinguish himself from "the kind of people [we] know" as drug researchers). Similarly, José Tisado, another participant, sat down in my office to begin an epidemiological survey that typically took an hour and a half to complete. As I opened the file containing the survey he asked, "This is the survey where you ask me if I share needles, right? I don't. Can I have my money now?" Through its at times obsessive focus on drug paraphernalia use (e.g., Feldman and Biernacki 1988), the very practice of social science research on drug use and HIV risk seems to send a message to participants that researchers are concerned about syringe sharing even to the exclusion of other features of their lives, habits, or structures of risk.

In some cases, researchers constitute an important point of contact between drug users and a public health apparatus bent on encouraging individuals to take personal responsibility for health and health care, particularly in the realm of behavioral health (Moore and Fraser 2006). The War on Drugs has intensified the criminalization of the minority poor and the transcarceration of the mentally ill (Mauer and Chesney-Lind 2002). These tendencies are exacerbated by the neoliberal withdrawal of resources from the inner city, leading to sharp decreases in the availability of publicly funded drug treatment programs. Structural forces such as these converge in ways that pressure interactions between ethnographers and research participants. When I interviewed drug users who expressed the desire to stop using drugs or even just get a firmer grip on their habits, I felt overwhelmed by the extent of their troubles, many of which far exceeded their drug use (homelessness, for example, or negotiating abusive relationships). My own resources—phone numbers of treatment programs that inevitably led to waiting lists, referrals to food pantries that required a permanent mailing address to confirm eligibility—seemed sorely inadequate to meet the needs of those I interviewed in any significant way.

In light of these intense structural contradictions, the principles and pragmatics of harm reduction seemed to offer little consolation.[8] This made it all the stranger when IDUs I interviewed responded to me, often before I even began to ask questions, as though I were the figure to whom they would be accountable for demonstrating adherence to these principles. An interview with George Davis, a middle-aged African American gentleman who had been using heroin and cocaine for at least three decades,

---

8. Similarly, the syringe exchange workers portrayed in Chapter 6 are mandated by state law to offer clients referrals to drug treatment programs, a system where waiting lists for publicly funded treatment beds can be months long. Given the frequent upheavals in users' lives, providers' ability to locate a user in that time frame are extremely slim.

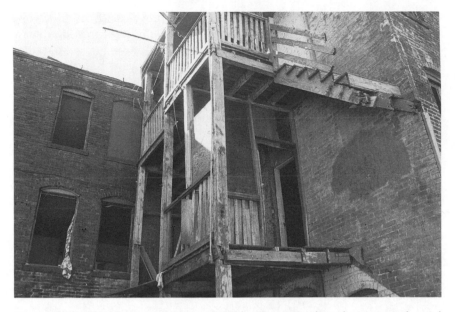

Many of Thornton's tenements, constructed to house workers during its industrial heyday, are now crumbling. *(Photograph courtesy of Amanda Quinby.)*

illustrated the strength of these expectations. Reminiscing about the partying he did "back in the day," he interrupted himself to declare that he never shared syringes. He told me that he always knew about blood, "that blood is a microscopic thing. . . . Because even though you don't see no blood in there, that's what's got a lot of people fucked up, so to speak. They don't see no blood up in there [in the tube of the syringe], they washed it out with water, they thinkin' it was clean. No sirree Bob." He articulates the kind of common sense public health prevention educators dream about, a common sense that endorses no syringe sharing among users: "All you have to do is just get your own set of works, and keep 'em. Don't share with nobody. If somebody want to use your works, don't let 'em use 'em, even if they do say, 'Well, I got bleach.' No. You don't do that. Get your own damn works, man. That's how I been doing it for years. I never shared with nobody, even back in the day." Does such a common sense really exist among IDUs, or did Davis feel compelled to say this because I was interviewing him for an HIV prevention study? Leshawna Bailey, a former heroin user and syringe exchange activist, felt that the "common sense" articulated by Davis was in fact already an internalized norm among IDUs:

> I'm just saying as a recovering addict, as someone who used to shoot dope, and it wasn't too long ago, that the education is out

there, so common sense will tell you, [if] you gonna use a used syringe, then you would bleach it out. Because common sense is out there. So [if] you can't get access to a clean syringe, you definitely can get free access to bleach kits and you can go find bleach in a cabinet. And I have yet to find a used syringe or buy a used syringe and not bleach it out.

This participant offered her own drug-using behavior as a sterling example of the "common sense" out there among drug users in general. In setting her own behavior as representative, Bailey constitutes herself as an ethical subject who adheres to what she assumed I valued and sought to document: responsible adherence to harm reduction behavior.[9] As Dave Wood insisted, "I don't play that"—indicating a principled refusal to share syringes that he assumed to be the focus of our in-depth interview. Such assertions are efforts to establish an ethical position for the self that adheres to the harm reduction standards that participants believe researchers hold. Many of those we spoke with in the Syringe Access study described similar levels of adherence to harm reduction prescriptions. While people's injection practices certainly did not uniformly match these norms, I heard articulations of these norms from both those who acted on them and those who failed to do so.

I also observed users who seized on a particular action that they believed would correspond with the normative practices of harm reduction. During drug use observations, participants' actions seemed to illustrate a particular norm or set of norms that they assumed I was trying to document.[10] For example, when I observed two African American friends sharing a bag of heroin, each used their own syringe while they shared a cooker[11] and the bag of heroin. Because Frank Barton was too self-conscious to inject himself in front of an observer, his friend Harold

9. See Moore and Fraser 2006 for a discussion of the ways in which this kind of "neoliberal subjectivity" (3038) may be empowering for people who occupy marginalized positions in society.

10. To gather detailed information about actual drug use practices that may exceed or contradict reported behavior, the Syringe Access study included direct observation of injection drug use with participants (see Singer et al. 2000 for further methodological details). In each of the three research sites, these activities included an ethnographer, usually accompanied by an outreach worker, working from a written interview guide containing a space in which to diagram the location of participants and paraphernalia. As the site ethnographer for Thornton, I invited participants to do a drug use observation only after they had already completed several other activities with me, such as the lengthy epidemiological survey and an in-depth interview.

11. A cooker is any small container—a bottle cap, spoon, or the concave bottom of a soda can—used to mix powdered heroin with water; it is called a cooker because generally heat is applied to the bottom using a lighter.

Moore did it for him. In this case it was the water that Moore decided was important. Barton picked up a plastic cup off his dresser and handed it to Moore to use to mix up the dope. Harold looked at the water skeptically and asked if it was new. Barton said, "Coulda swore I just put this water in this cup." But Moore demurred, saying petulantly, "Well, I didn't see you."

"Watch me," Barton replied as he got up to go into the kitchen.

"I'm watching you now," said Moore as Barton elaborately tossed the water down the sink and refilled the cup from the tap. They were both laughing as I asked if they always bickered like that. Moore said, "I have to be very careful. Ain't going to pass nothing on to nobody. You know what I mean? . . . I make sure I bleach; today I didn't have no bleach, but normally I do that. And when I get through with my tools, I put 'em in a bag and go up to [the Waterford exchange ten miles away] and exchange it for brand new ones." Yet at the end of this injection session Barton rinsed his own syringe with water from the same cup Moore drew from and used no bleach to clean it. Meanwhile Moore recapped his syringe without rinsing it. By drawing up into his syringe water that had been used by another possibly HIV-infected syringe, Barton exposed himself to the possibility of transmitting HIV to his own syringe.[12]

In another instance, Juan Solano, a middle-aged Puerto Rican heroin user, squatted in the woods outside an apartment building to prepare his dose with the help of a younger friend, Teddy Montoya. As I closely observed and took notes on his procedures, Solano took a piece of paper to use as a table of sorts because he did not want to put his supplies right on the ground. He pulled his syringe out of his pocket, and Montoya gave him a bleach kit containing water, cooker, and bleach. He opened the water bottle, poured a little in the cap, and put it on the paper. He pulled a minuscule glassine bag from his pocket and tore it open with his teeth after trying and failing to open it with his fingers. Carefully drying the open bag on his jeans so that none of the powder would stick to the moisture, Solano sprinkled the heroin into the bottle-top cooker and used the syringe to squirt water from the bottle in the bleach kit into the cooker to dissolve the heroin.

Solano asked Montoya for a piece of cotton—somehow in the course of mixing up his drugs they had lost the cotton that came in the bleach kit, or it was lost earlier. (A filter prevents particulates that remain in the heroin-water mixture from being drawn up into the syringe.) Montoya pulled a thread off his shirt, washed his hands using another water bottle, and

---

12. Mark Davis and Tim Rhodes (2004) describe the idea of "unseen blood" proposed to IDUs in interviews to be "a new and unsettling idea, partly because it undermined blood management" practices based on what the authors described as "altruistic conduct," and what I consider harm reduction norms.

made a little ball with the thread. He handed the ball to Solano to use as a filter for drawing up the heroin-water mixture, but Solano said, "I want to do it with my own fingers," and proceeded to repeat the whole procedure, washing his hands and then the thread ball with water before dropping it into the cooker. In this case, Solano seized on a particular aspect of the injection process—injecting with a clean cotton filter—as the part to be especially concerned about, perhaps because of fears of hepatitis or "cotton fever." Solano was worried enough about the status of the cotton to argue about it, yet when I asked if his syringe was new, he reported that it was "second used. . . . I didn't use it. A friend of mine did."

While these participants clearly espouse some harm reduction norms, their verbal presentations differ from their actual performances during ethnographic observations ("I make sure I bleach; today I didn't have no bleach, but normally I do that"). While drug users endorse and even practice harm reduction norms, their ambivalent willingness to occupy the risk categories created by public health discourse can be seen in their uneven adoption of and resistance to certain harm reduction norms. For example, despite IDUs' frequent statements to me about cleaning syringes with bleach, field observations in both Massachusetts and Connecticut have shown that bleaching is not the norm among drug injectors, as evidenced by the unopened miniature bleach bottles that littered outdoor injection sites we surveyed. The uptake of bleach has been reluctant, and the scientific evidence that it works equivocal (Bourgois 2002). As well, many pragmatic factors shape their ability to adhere to these norms (Buchanan et al. 2002).

In addition to providing empirical evidence of "risk," ethnographic encounters reveal the work participants do to (re)position themselves as ethical subjects on their own terms. Users are aware that they are under scrutiny, that data gathered about their experiences will be used in calculations of health and risk that correspond to moral worth. Carrying out state-funded drug research thus places ethnographers and outreach workers in the position of *representing* to IDUs the goals of HIV risk reduction: "don't share syringes, clean your works." Given how rooted public health and substance abuse regimes are in imbuing certain forms of behavior with moral value (Petersen and Lupton 1996), a gap opens between those who deliver prescriptive messages and those who are "targets" of intervention. The moral value associated with abstinence under the War on Drugs is gradually being replaced by a neoliberal emphasis on individual responsibility for health and HIV prevention that dovetails conveniently with notions of individual "empowerment" in harm reduction (Moore and Fraser 2006). The ensuing contradictions for harm reduction organizations, portrayed in the following chapter, reflect the experiences of community health outreach programs discussed in Part I. Concepts of risk figure largely in these processes.

Drug Research and the Proliferation of Risk

Applied social research on drug use and HIV is the process of learning to see and then represent degrees of risk. In a paper about drug users' practices of containing visible and invisible blood during injection, Mark Davis and Tim Rhodes (2004) comment on the disciplinary effect of the structured public health interview between researcher and IDU in which "blood literally comes into view" (380) as a representation of HIV risk. Similarly, training outreach workers and ethnographers to do research on HIV transmission among IDUs entails helping them learn to *see* the risk that is subsequently quantified in self-report surveys. "Follow the blood," a co-investigator on the Syringe Access project used to say, from syringe to water to cooker to syringe to vein. HIV prevention educators and harm reduction workers take part in the proliferation of risk every time they "educate" users that water touched by a used syringe is potentially contaminated and therefore must be treated as if it *were* contaminated. Ethnographers and other drug researchers then document and quantify this proliferating risk that is elicited from IDUs first by harm reduction educators and then by the "risk assessment" interview.

Active drug users' perceptions of themselves as being *at risk* for HIV are shaped in part by epidemiological and ethnographic findings on HIV transmission that undergird scientific constructions of risk. These constructions contribute to people's perceptions and behaviors in ways unanticipated by researchers and harm reduction advocates. In the Syringe Access project this was illustrated by the Syringe Acquisition Interview (SAI), in which an ethnographer accompanies a participant as she procures syringes from her usual sources in order to learn where and how IDUs acquire syringes, and to collect syringes being sold on the street for laboratory testing. We found that participants used a variety of terms to rate the degree of risk represented by a given syringe (Eiserman et al. 2003). A diabetic might sell a syringe after using it to inject himself with insulin; heroin users regarded this form of "skin popping" as fairly safe in terms of HIV risk and rated diabetics as preferable to other drug users or street sellers as syringe providers (Stopka et al. 2003). Julie Eiserman and colleagues identified "emic" categories of risk used to describe syringes purchased on the street (2003). The harm reduction norm of "always use a new/clean syringe every time you inject" was invoked by drug users even when previously used syringes were purchased. Depending on *who* used it in *what* manner, a participant might rate a given syringe as "new" rather than used and calculate the degree of risk as less rather than more.

Harm reduction norms and techniques have made new syringes seem "safer" than old ones, to such an extent that users will even insist that a clearly used syringe is actually new in order to occupy the position of an ethical user concerned with protecting their own and others' health. A syringe cleaned with bleach, considered *as safe as* a new syringe, may now be called "new." Even when confronted with evidence that the syringe was used, a participant might continue to insist that it was new. For example, in one SAI, Doug Reaves disappeared into an apartment building a few blocks from where he and I had met. He returned a few minutes later to report that he had bought two syringes for eight dollars from Lonny, a heroin user and diabetic whom I later came to know as a syringe seller. When I asked Reaves during the subsequent interview whether the syringes he bought from Lonny were new or used, he reported that the syringes "look new to me." When I later examined one of the syringes, however, I found blood congealed in its tip, clearly indicating that it was used. Another part of the SAI asked participants to describe their regular syringe-purchasing habits. In this section of the interview, Reaves reported that he never bought used syringes. I asked what he would do if he suspected that his regular syringe source was selling him a used syringe, and he said, "I give it back." These assertions were not uncommon. When I asked Sam Sullivan, another participant, at the end of an SAI if he had ever bought used syringes, he said, "Only once." Earlier in the interview, however, he talked about crisis moments when his usual source was unavailable, and he would look everywhere, hoping to find a syringe on the street or in the park.

> Sam: I don't have any choice. I go to the park and look around to see if I can find any of my syringes there.
> Susan: How will you know they are yours?
> Sam: Nobody hides their syringes where anybody else does. Mine, I put under a tree, covered with a log. If that log has been moved, I know someone took my syringes.
> Susan: How long will you wait for her?
> Sam: I'll wait a little while. The most I will wait for a person is an hour. After that hour, forget it. Either that or I try to buy it off of somebody else.

When directly queried, users seek to maintain the position that they adhere to harm reduction norms by "never" sharing syringes or purchasing used syringes. When Sullivan described his daily routine, however, it became clear that when circumstances forced him to do so, he relied on syringes used by others first, or even his own that he had stashed in a public location.[13]

---

13. Users would stash syringes in places such as parks or out-of-the-way outdoor injection sites because of paraphernalia laws that criminalized possession of a syringe without a doctor's prescription (Martinez et al. 2007). Being arrested for drug possession while also carrying a (new or used) syringe meant an additional felony charge. In cities with syringe exchange programs, IDUs must produce a membership card to the arresting officer to avoid such charges. See the Landry case, described in note 15 of Chapter 6.

Using ethnographic and epidemiological research, researchers create the terms through which using a syringe that someone else has used first or using a syringe of indeterminate status is understood as a "risky" practice. The survey instruments we use to monitor risk then enforce the terms of what counts as risky behavior. Those terms are behaviorally but also *morally* defined (Berger 2004): If you shoot drugs, do you share syringes? How many people do you share with? If you have sex, do you wear a condom? How often? Despite their painstakingly neutral phrasing, these questions always carry moral valuations. Given this, we can interpret statements such as "We always use bleach!" as strategically useful constructions that assert users' ethical personhood in the face of their reduction to mere membership in an epidemiological category.

Elaborations of risk—whether produced by epidemiologists, actuaries, or statisticians—call for ever-expanding regimes of vigilance, surveillance, and control (Castel 1991; Miller 2001b). "By focusing not on individuals but on factors of risk, on statistical correlations of heterogeneous elements, the experts have multiplied the possibilities for preventive intervention" (Petersen 1997, 193). Though discourses of harm reduction emerged from grassroots organizing by current and former drug users, they dovetail with neoliberal surveillance regimes that encourage personal responsibility for health (Fischer et al. 2004; Moore and Fraser 2006). The responsibilization of people who use drugs can be glimpsed in an ethical dilemma sometimes presented as a litmus test to new or would-be drug researchers: "You're observing an HIV-discordant pair about to get high together. They have only one syringe between them. What do you do?" The dilemma pits the researcher's ethical obligation of beneficence against that of protecting confidentiality. Some opt for protecting the confidentiality of the HIV-positive individual because, among other things, it supports their own goal of being able to continue doing research. This solution transfers responsibility for the interaction to each individual participating in it, as the observer may think, "Well, he *should* be protecting himself anyway!"

In "Addiction Markets: The Case of High-Dose Buprenorphine in France," Anne Lovell argues that French harm reduction has "evolved into a highly individualized set of bodily practices and discourses that are resonant with the individually focused 'new public health' (Petersen and Lupton 1996), which locates responsibility in the lifestyle of the individual as purely an individual decision" (2006, 161). Lovell notes that the drug user constituted by harm reduction discourse is rendered not simply a "target" of intervention but an individual "decision maker who rank-orders his or her own practices in terms of the level of risk he or she 'chooses' (to inject 'safely' rather than to stop injecting, to sniff rather than inject, to use 'soft' drugs rather than 'hard,' and so on)" (2006, 161). This move effectively disembeds risk from the structural conditions that produced it, locating harm as an individual matter to be dealt with privately and attributing moral value to certain risk-related decisions but not others.

Specifying Identities

Studies seeking to understand institutional responses to drug use often present drug users as more similar to than different from consumers of other products (e.g., Glick Schiller, Crystal, and Lewellen 1994; Storper 2000; O'Malley 1999). Indeed, the generic term *user* appears throughout public health and harm reduction literature, evoking a widespread tendency to refer to people as "users" to indicate their relationship to some form of technology—computers, automatic teller machines (ATMs), surveillance cameras, and so on (Oudshoorn and Pinch 2003). Referring to IDUs as "users" indicates a similar consumer relationship to both their drug of choice and the technology of ingesting it (syringes, pipes). Elizabeth Ettore argues that "users are seen as consumers of drugs that become intertwined with the cultures of everyday life" (2004, 328). This counters the persistent tendency to think of drug use as all-consuming, and addiction as subsuming all other activities. At the same time, this phrase linguistically highlights a single aspect of a person's existence: her consumption of illicit drugs, and even (in the label *IDU*) her method of use (injection). This label collapses the different types of drugs a user might inject (Bourgois and Bruneau 2000), as well as the different types of relationships someone might have with her drug of choice, ranging from abject addiction to casual use (Duff 2004). With these limitations and elisions firmly in mind, I continue to rely on the terms *user* and *IDU* for convenience, and to signal the ambivalent possibilities and harms entailed in recognizing the subject-forming potential of habitual drug consumption.

Within this overarching category of "user," detailed ethnographic studies have created ever-narrower specifications based on both behaviors and identities—we now have categories for, and perhaps even mental images of, "inner-city drug-using Puerto Ricans," "homeless injection drug users," "drug-injecting youth," "substance-abusing victims of domestic violence," and so on. While the proliferation of highly differentiated subpopulations has furthered the development of ever more appropriate, culturally sensitive, and effective interventions, these behavioral categories must also be recognized as new *categories for governing* that did not exist before the research. Insofar as the provision of specialized services (e.g., shelters for drug-using women involved in violent relationships) makes people newly subject to state and other forms of authority, these programs can be seen as techniques of governing applied to the new populations delineated by research (Rose 1999).

While *IDU* emerged as a behavior-based population designation for researchers and service providers alike, ethnographic interviews with drug users emphasize that, in contrast, IDUs identify along a variety of dimensions—as women, as Puerto Rican, as mothers, as truck drivers. Their self-conception may or may not revolve around their externally identified "risk category." Some clearly do inhabit the category to which they are assigned, like the woman who said, "Why should I be afraid to use the [syringe exchange] van? This is who I am." Others prioritize their families, jobs, or marriages above their drug habit (Agar 2002), while for still others, feeling trapped in an abusive relationship is an even more significant problem than their addiction.

Social relationships also seem to influence users' conceptualizations of risk. For example, Tony Edwards, an African American participant, reported that his favorite syringe source of those we visited in an SAI was "the one on [St. Mark's] Avenue. Sometimes when you ask someone [to sell you a syringe], if they're in a bad mood or something, they don't want to give it to you. [This guy,] he's not like that." Edwards also preferred this seller because "he don't give you a hard time. A lot of these other guys want to argue with you about the price." Whether syringes are new or used seemed less important to Edwards than their availability, which may be subject to the seller's mood as well as the price.

When asked directly, Edwards reported that he never, or seldom, bought used syringes, yet all three sellers we visited during our interview sold us used syringes. In fact, the syringe he obtained from the seller he deemed the best and most reliable was also the most clearly used syringe, with all numbers and lettering worn off. As we were driving around later discussing it with two of his friends, Edwards seemed unconcerned about the condition of this latter syringe. When I asked what he would do if he had bought it for his own use, he said that he would be sure to clean it. "How?" I asked. He answered, "By running it under water." One of Edwards's friends admonished him at this point that water was not enough to keep you from getting HIV or hepatitis C and instructed him to use bleach—another example of performing harm reduction norms, as well as the dissemination of those norms among peers who are willing to correct each other on their performances.

In another SAI, José Fernandez, a young Puerto Rican heroin user, brought me to three different syringe sellers. One of them, Prieto, sold a syringe that Fernandez reported to me was "new" but clearly appeared used (the plunger cap was missing, and the tip of the plunger was broken just beneath the rubber stopper). He said that he paid three dollars for the syringe. When I asked Fernandez which of the three sellers we visited that day was his preferred source, he chose Prieto "because he's a nice guy, and he always has some. You know when you go up to him, you sure you're going to get it." Though we also visited another seller who Fernandez reported is usually available and "always has" new syringes, Fernandez preferred to go to Prieto because he knows him and likes him. But in this instance at least, Prieto sold Fernandez a used syringe at the price of a new syringe. At other moments, however, social relations among users and between users and syringe providers may function as exclusionary mechanisms directing users' preferences. For example, Joanna Morgan, a white female user I interviewed, described a shooting gallery near one of her regular syringe sources. She said that she had never been in the gallery "because I think it's mainly Spanish [meaning Latino] and it's mainly men so I don't go in it." Other, more typically recognized features of identity such as gender and ethnicity limit her decisions about where to inject and where to get her syringes. Among all those I interviewed, however, access to sterile syringes was overwhelmingly limited by their extreme poverty and by the political-economic situation (discussed further in Chapter 6) criminalizing the possession of syringes without a prescription and limiting the availability of syringe exchange in Thornton. These laws, in place until at least 2006, drove up costs of syringes purchased on the street (up to five dollars a syringe at a time when individual bags of heroin were selling for ten dollars and a bundle, or ten bags, for fifty dollars). In response, IDUs would take measures that seemed desperate, such as stashing syringes in public areas or digging up syringes buried in dirt to reuse them after a quick rinse. Chapter 6 details efforts by harm reduction activists to bring syringe exchange to Thornton to mitigate these harms; however, syringes were decriminalized before activists won their campaign, allowing pharmacies to sell them over the counter without a prescription.

Even as they critique the classificatory scheme that designates nonmedical drug users as *criminals*, and medical users as *patients* suffering from a disease, ethnographic contributions to epidemiological risk calculations help problematize drug use as a health issue amenable to public health solutions. As discussed further in Chapter 6, an overarching governing mentality in U.S. drug policy has persistently set criminal justice over and against medicine (Campbell 2000). The oppositional logic of crime versus disease positions "harm reduction," the discursive object of this chapter, as a third alternative (Marlatt 1996). Consisting of a pragmatic set of discursive and material practices drafted to recognize the limits of behaviorism for achieving abstinence, harm reduction discourse acknowledges the incremental nature of behavioral change and constructs addiction as a chronic condition of relapse and recovery.

As a mode of knowledge production designed, at least in part, to aid the management of troublesome populations, ethnographic research on drug use partakes of a regime of truth closely related to the desire to intervene (Dean 1999). I argue that drug ethnographers' subjects have largely been assimilated to the project of risk and harm reduction, and I ask: What are the structural and discursive conditions that have produced the subjects of drug ethnography today? How does combining ethnographic research with public health prevention messages affect ethnographic methodology?

Is ethnography an adjunct to a public health delivery system, where ethnographers are not simply documenting subcultural practices but are harnessed to a state bent on surveilling behaviors emerging in so-called hidden populations? Epidemiological notions of risk groups serve as a classificatory scheme for categorizing populations on the basis of behavior, individualizing harm and personalizing prevention (Petersen and Lupton 1996; Lupton 1999).

James Scott (1998) argues that state-funded representations of complex and variable communities are always, of necessity, reductions of complexity. "State agents," he writes, "have no interest . . . in describing an entire social reality. . . . Their abstractions and simplifications are disciplined by a small number of objectives" (23)—in this case, the desire to minimize the spread of infectious disease among drug users, to encourage the "responsibilization" (Fischer and Poland 1998) of drug users for risk reduction behavior, or to reduce the harm of drug use.

At the same time, official categorizations of drug users as a deviant population have been challenged and eroded by new social movements oriented toward health (Valverde 1998). Drug ethnographers, activists, and community health workers have served as relays for creating, transmitting, and enforcing harm reduction norms in the field. Researchers shaped both the perception and practice of harm reduction norms at institutional and individual levels (Campbell and Shaw 2008). Researchers adopted and embodied harm reduction values, even as IDUs, far from endorsing oppositional stances toward public health authority figures, incorporated the languages and ethical positions of those who have studied them. As service delivery and surveillance converge, new ethical subject-positions are created for researchers and subjects alike.

As the category of *IDU* expands to incorporate harm reduction behaviors and norms, it is a an example of a behavior-based identity category that has taken on new ethical meanings at the same time as other aspects of identity—such as gender, ethnicity, or profession—recede from view. Simultaneously, the relational, structural, and contextual factors that ethnographers set out to clarify (Schoepf 2001) have proven difficult to measure and even harder to change. Since little ethnographic research has shown that drug users exclusively ground their identities in their drug of choice or mode of drug delivery, I highlight the discursive means through which the reduction of diverse groups of people to IDUs takes place. At the same time, this analysis is inescapably subject to the same criticism.

Anthropological research can counter this process by contributing nonreductive accounts of personhood and the multiple ways in which people exceed the categories to which their behaviors are assigned by techniques of governance (e.g., Bourgois 2009; Garcia 2010). As ethnographic work is picked up and reproduced in ways beyond our control, drug ethnography contributes to the formation and solidification of behavior-based population categories that ultimately exclude the very holistic details that we, as anthropologists, have argued are crucial to health. The danger is that through earnest efforts to identify and reduce the risk of HIV transmission among drug users—and to avoid furthering the stigmatization of particular ethnic and social groups—we will end up foreclosing the very spaces of possibility for personhood that are crucial to successful HIV prevention efforts, which take account of cultural context. By focusing on behavioral risk to the exclusion of social, cultural, and structural contexts, we run the risk of eviscerating the libratory possibilities of a prevention movement that is also simultaneously a movement for social justice.

6

Syringe Exchange as a Practice of Governing

Despite widespread evidence of their effectiveness in reducing the spread of HIV among injection drug users (IDUs), syringe exchange programs (SEPs), which provide sterile syringes to IDUs in return for used ones, remain controversial. As perhaps the most widely practiced innovation of the harm reduction movement, SEPs act on users' actions by providing them the means to use a sterile syringe for every injection. To accomplish this, SEPs across the United States use techniques ranging from strictly enforced one-for-one exchange to encouraging secondary exchange, in which individual members collect syringes from their contacts and exchange them at the SEP in bulk. In an effort to address SEP opponents' fears of discarded syringes and needle sticks by "the innocent" (archetypically, children in a playground), few programs allow syringe distribution without any required exchange of used syringes. These variations in policy both shape the local ecology of HIV risk and manifest collective struggles over how to manage and protect the public's health. The question of who makes up the public whose health is threatened—people addicted to drugs who risk HIV infection as they inject, or "innocent" children in a city playground—is a key component of these struggles.

These debates reveal schisms and conflicts over the proper role of government, the importance of personal responsibility in individual conduct, and who counts as a citizen or a member of a community. As they seek to regulate drug users' practices and reduce the physical and social harm caused by illicit and injection drug use, SEPs are engaged in projects of governance similar to those described in Part I. As more-or-less developed organizational outgrowths of an earlier social movement (harm reduction), SEPs work to shape the behavior of IDUs according to the harm reduction norms described in the previous chapter (e.g., use a sterile syringe every time you inject). At the same time, SEPs support the state's larger goal of reducing drug use by providing what advocates often referred to as a "continuum of care." In Massachusetts, the law authorizing state-funded syringe exchange mandates that SEPs make every effort to place IDUs who visit the exchange in drug treatment programs—a mandate that stands in contrast to a harm reduction orientation that "meets users where they're at" and encourages moderation rather than abstinence from drug use (O'Hare et al. 1992; Small et al. 2010). Harm reduction programs struggle with adopting neoliberal norms of individual responsibility while they simultaneously maintain larger critiques of authoritarian approaches to drug use (Rothschild 1998; Roe 2005). SEP advocates and staff aim to provide IDUs with the tools (syringes) they can use to avoid HIV infection and to meet a broad range of other needs as well, such as housing, food, and domestic violence intervention. Like the Community Health Advocate (CHA) program portrayed in Part I, SEPs, as grassroots organizations responding to the concerns of marginalized groups, serve as a technology for both governing drug users and advancing their interests.

As they work to protect the health and represent the interests of a stigmatized population, SEPs, often in partnership with AIDS service organizations and drug treatment programs, seek to expand the definition of who counts as a citizen and a member of "the public" (Shaw 2006). At the same time, SEPs regulate the behavior of an unruly population at the level of the micropractices of drug use (e.g., injection techniques and paraphernalia). In examining SEPs as a technology of government, we can begin to pry apart the regimes of knowledge and practice that shape these programs and their effects on individuals and collectivities. I begin by looking at the racialized and economic assumptions through which drug users—particularly urban, minority IDUs—are constructed as less than full citizens because of their dependency on illicit drugs. As organizations developed by former and sometimes even current drug users, SEPs take part in the liberatory discourse of community health, mobilizing a collective identity in order to make claims on the state and on health care providers. This mobilization is accompanied by efforts to destigmatize a highly stigmatized identity (Small et al. 2010). SEPs become more institutionalized, however, as they win funding and contracts from state public health agencies and local governments. SEPs are thereby subject to demands of accountability similar to those of the community health programs described in Part I. Last, I discuss the governing mentalities (Campbell 2000) of SEPs as they work to produce certain subjectivities among their IDU clients.[1] These harm reduction mentalities aim to reform drug user conduct and bring IDUs into the body politic as clients, if not citizens, by engaging them in a broader continuum of care aimed at eliminating drug use by entering drug users into treatment programs. Yet by building on a history of drug user and HIV activism, SEPs also challenge the stigmatization of drug users as dependents who are disabled by addiction, organizing a range of resources and services to diverse groups of drug users (e.g., Henman et al. 1998).

Practicing Harm Reduction in Hard Times

The harm reduction framework that orients the work of many SEPs in the United States and abroad is characterized by a nonjudgmental attitude toward drug users that views each individual as worthwhile and valuable, if beset by the problems that accompany addiction (Marlatt 1996). A counselor at a Thornton drop-in center for active drug users summed up the harm reduction mentality this way: "Our primary purpose is to serve the intravenous drug users. We use a harm reduction strategy, we don't tell them to stop, we just tell them if you're gonna use, try not to harm yourself, here is how you can use safely, but if you want to stop, this is what we can provide for you." Another substance abuse counselor emphasized, "We gotta help these people. They're human beings like us." Taking a nonjudgmental approach allows harm reduction programs to establish relationships with members of a population often deemed "hard to reach" by service providers and to link users with HIV prevention and drug treatment services they might otherwise avoid. A Thornton public health official who was a supporter of syringe exchange described a harm reduction approach to injection drug use that incorporates primary health care, a disease model of substance abuse, syringe exchange, and access to drug treatment:

> Well, I guess I look at primary health care as a prevention-intervention strategy, so I think injection drug users need to have primary health care as a basic service. The other public health strategy, to come back to [your question on] needle exchange—that is another primary health care strategy that injection drug users need to

---

1. Nancy Campbell observes, "Although figurative in nature, [governing mentalities] are materialized in institutions, policy-making cultures, and bureaucratic-administrative programs and procedures. Governing mentalities derive their power to compel from both symbolic and material registers" (2000, 50). As explored in Chapter 5, SEPs and harm reduction organizations, in their interactions with IDUs, both depend on and produce an at-risk subjectivity that proactively works to mitigate risk and harm by adhering to harm reduction norms, reducing drug consumption, and using wraparound services including drug treatment to escape addiction altogether.

have. [There's] [t]he whole issue around seeing injection drug use and substance abuse as a disease, an addiction, versus a punitive [approach], as if people are born wanting to be injection drug users. . . . So, the needs are around, viewing substance abuse as a disease, getting people into primary health care, getting them what they need in terms of needle exchange, getting individuals what they need as far as support from the community and family. There are layers and layers probably, but primarily it's prevention/intervention for me; it's primary health care and the whole issue of harm reduction and helping people to get into treatment.

As discussed in greater detail in Chapter 5, at the same time that they maintain a pragmatic attitude toward addiction, harm reduction programs may also incorporate a neoliberal emphasis on personal responsibility for health (Moore and Fraser 2006), as seen in this excerpt from the *Controlled Substance Field Manual*, 2000 edition, a copy of which was given to me by Chris Collins from the Highpoint program. The manual, designed by the Massachusetts Criminal Justice Training Council, introduces police officers to SEPs this way:

> There are currently four department [of public health–]funded needle exchange programs operating in Massachusetts located in Boston, Cambridge, [Waterford,] and Provincetown. The programs strive to create an atmosphere that encourages compassion, self-respect and positive action within the injection drug using (IDU) community. Participants are encouraged to take responsibility for their lifestyle choices and are assisted in identifying interventions that could be of help. The creation and implementation of this environment and attitude will ultimately help to slow the spread of HIV infection within [the] IDU community. (2000, 126)

It is noteworthy that the audience for this articulation of what Akhil Gupta and Aradhana Sharma would call "the concerns with empowerment and self-help characteristic of neoliberal governmentality" (2006, 278) was police officers, who were perhaps thought to be more receptive to an ideology of self-help ("take responsibility for their lifestyle choices") than to other, antiauthoritarian aspects of harm reduction (Roe 2005). Harm reduction norms emphasizing individual responsibility for health also focus on the importance of self-regulation for health, in the form of knowing one's limits (Duff 2004) or, in the words of one needle exchange worker, "too much for my own good." Many harm reduction advocates locate the source of the pain and suffering that surround illicit drug use in the social structures associated with the criminalization of using certain substances (or "status behaviors"; see Buchanan et al. 2002); in contrast, behavior-based interventions targeted to the individual drug user implicitly place responsibility on the individual user herself.

As discussed in Chapter 3, ideologies of personal responsibility broadly support economic expressions of neoliberalism such as the shrinking welfare state (Harvey 2005). Even when established and supported by the state, the SEPs I studied faced the difficult combination of constantly decreasing budgets and ever-expanding caseloads, as word of the resources they offer spread among drug users. In a 2004 meeting of Connecticut SEPs, the head of a Hartford program said that his organization was trying to expand its search for financial support beyond the state department of public health because that funding was so capricious and unreliable—at that time, supporting only two days of syringe exchange per week. One strategy his organization, WeCare, developed was to collaborate on research projects with nearby universities to cover staff salaries and supplies for the rest of the week. They were not always successful, however, and the previous year WeCare had had to cut back services to only four days a week because of budget cuts. They were currently struggling to maintain service five days a week. Another SEP director remarked that Connecticut SEPs were totally discouraged and "disempowered" as they faced seemingly inevitable budget cuts, regardless of advocates' protests. The "new market-oriented state" (Biehl 2007, 11) imposes a logic of both scarcity (in shrinking public dollars) and entrepreneurialism; as one AIDS service organization director responded, "What you have to do is diversify your funding sources."

An AIDS lobbyist at the meeting reported that over the last three years state support for SEPs declined from $425,000 to $316,000. The biggest cut came two years earlier, a 17 percent reduction in funding. When I asked what such cuts meant, concretely, another staff member explained that they were forced to give drug users fewer alcohol preps (suggested for cleaning the injection site before injecting) and fewer cookers (used to mix heroin with water before injection) and to make other reductions in supplies. In an in-depth interview, another SEP director reported, "We really did run out of syringes at one point" as a result of budget cuts. The increasing hegemony of individualizing neoliberal ideologies combined with ever more constrained funding environments push even programs with the most comprehensive cultural critiques to bend toward individual-level prevention interventions, balancing population-based health promotion with beliefs about individual responsibility for health (Moore and Fraser 2006).

Crime versus Disease: Framing Local Ambivalence around Syringe Exchange

Addiction generally, and SEPs in particular, pose unique challenges to local and broader conceptions of how to govern and promote the public health. How are drug users categorized, as sick or dangerous? What forms of entitlement do states and communities grant these sick or dangerous members? Why might criminals or clients be entitled to syringes but not health care? Why does obtaining an HIV infection qualify a criminal or client for care (Biehl 2007)? What kinds of care can be given, by whom, and for how long?[2] Administrators and elected officials struggle over the answers to these and myriad related questions as they make and contest decisions around local health policies such as syringe exchange.

Conflicting social constructions of IDUs set in motion the ambivalent state support for SEPs discussed in this chapter. From the perspective of law enforcement, and many lawmakers on both state and local levels, IDUs present a threat to be handled through the criminal justice system. Their addiction signifies lawlessness and lack of control. In contrast, from the perspective of the Massachusetts Department of Public Health, IDUs are members of the body politic in need of behavioral treatment and management. Both these constructions hinge on the helplessness of users in the face of their addiction. Like the women on welfare in Part I, dependence (in this case, on a needle or an illegal drug) constrains IDUs' ability to be regarded as and to occupy the role of citizens.

For the general public as well as among drug users, a special stigma is attached to the use of needles as a powerful symbol of both risk and dependency. For example, George Davis, the heroin user we met in Chapter 5, explained, "I think that IV users are treated differently, because they seem like a lower, like trash. You got a dude that smokes crack, and they cool. The dealer, he'll sell you something, you're cool. . . . But a man that shoots dope, he's the lowest form. 'Oh, he do dope!'" Advanced marginalization and shrinking public budgets for prevention shape the social, political, and ecological context of HIV infections among IDUs, leading to the social and discursive construction of drug users as a population that is both "at risk" for HIV infection and a potential threat to "the public." Public contestation over syringe exchange is thus inflamed by both the actual risk for HIV among these marginalized groups and the fear and stigma that result from the increased risk and incidence of infection.

The "crime" and "disease" frames for political discourse on drug use outlined by Nancy Campbell (2000, 45) set the terms in which local and national political conflict over SEPs takes place. Harm reduction and public health interventions such as SEP position IDUs as *clients* rather

---

2. Mark Donovan (1996) explores the discourses of innocence and deservingness that authorize and animate programs such as the federal Ryan White Care Act, which provides a range of benefits for people who qualify with an AIDS diagnosis, including financial and case management assistance with housing, nutrition, medication, access to health care, and other services. A 2002 review of programs funded by the act found that "uninsured patients, women, people of color, and injection drug users waited much longer than others to receive new" highly active antiretroviral therapies under the provisions of the program (McKinney and Marconi 2002, 99).

than *criminals* by providing mental and primary health care (including, critically, HIV testing) in addition to sterile syringes and by working to medicalize addiction. Yet these constructions of drug users are countered by criminal justice interpretations that would punish users for breaking the law, like any other criminal. In contrast, harm reduction approaches to drug use instead invoke therapeutic frames of care and support (Carr 2009). Advocates for SEPs frequently speak of syringe exchange as just one element of a larger continuum of care. Parker, a white SEP worker at Highpoint, explained:

> [We have] needle exchange; it's a stationary exchange here in [Waterford]. Um, and we also offer, um, exchange within the city limits of [Waterford], not necessarily within this office. Like our outreach workers can exchange syringes within [Waterford] city limits. And [we offer] all sorts of ancillary [services]; we do referrals for treatment, detox. . . . We do HIV testing, counseling and testing; we do educational groups and individual educational and counseling sessions, mainly regarding HIV, safer injections, overdose prevention, uh, hepatitis C, vein care, safer sex, and so forth.

Similarly, an SEP in Hartford, Connecticut, sought additional funding in 2004 to offer "hepatitis services, primary health care screenings for diabetes, anti-pneumonia vaccines, anything that is health related." Such programs further the public health rationale for SEPs in addition to providing new, much-needed funding sources for cash-strapped programs that struggle against criminal justice constructions of drug users in their appeals for state and federal funding.[3]

Others, however, view supplying syringes to IDUs, even "in exchange for" used syringes, as tantamount to supporting an illegal activity. SEPs present health policy challenges unavoidably inflected by meanings of criminality and law and order. This was vividly illustrated in an exchange that took place at a meeting of the Thornton City Council's Public Safety Committee, ostensibly held to develop specific plans for SEPs in Thornton. In the ornate wood-trimmed council chambers, Frank Stein, an SEP advocate and former heroin user, asked Mary Norris, an undecided city councilor, what her main objection to SEPs was. "I think it's the ethical issue," she answered. "Can you say more about that?" Stein pressed. Norris said she thought it was wrong to support illegal behavior by providing people with free syringes. It was like giving them permission to use drugs. Another SEP advocate made an analogy to sexual morality, asking, "Do you think

---

3. In 1988, U.S. senator Jesse Helms sponsored legislation forbidding the use of federal funding for syringe exchange, a ban that lasted through both Democratic and Republican administrations until it was finally overturned in December 2009 (Egelko 2009).

giving your child a condom is giving them permission to have sex?" But Norris held her position, asking, "Why is it okay for the city to support an illegal activity?" When Stein responded sympathetically to this, commenting, "I used to think that myself," Norris changed tack by saying, "But we're doing it for free; that's the part I can't support."

Chris Collins, the Highpoint director, interjected, half joking, "Would you support the proposal if people were asked to pay for their needles?" Norris replied that she could not understand how IDUs could be unable to get the money to purchase needles on the black market if they have the money to pay for illegal drugs. Drawing a line from syringe access to biopolitics and value, a white woman in the audience stood up and said, "I'm sorry, I'm trying to wrap my mind around the idea that if you have money to pay for a clean needle then your life is worth more than the person who doesn't. It doesn't make sense to me." Her observation directs our attention to the life-and-death implications of a drug user's ability to purchase a sterile syringe for each injection of an illicit drug. By seeking to introduce SEPs as a state-sponsored HIV prevention technology, SEP advocates place the state in the gap between the ability to pay for a sterile syringe and the chance not to get infected with HIV. The previous commentator constructs an economically mediated kind of biocitizenship in which more affluent drug users, better able to protect their health by purchasing sterile syringes for each injection, are somehow more deserving of life than those less fortunate.[4]

Mary Norris, the undecided city councilor quoted earlier, was unable to read addiction or drug use as other than a law-and-order issue, in contrast to some SEP advocates who medicalize addiction as "a chronic relapsable condition." As Chris Collins explained on another occasion, at a community meeting on needle exchange in a predominantly African American neighborhood:

> The main thing my counselors talk about at the needle exchange program with their clients is how do you get clean. They're not all certified drug treatment counselors; some of them are, and some are on the way to being certified, but certainly most clients at a syringe exchange want to stop using drugs. The other important thing to realize is that addiction is a chronic relapsable condition. People get clean, but they frequently relapse, not just once but multiple times. And when they do, they're at high risk of contracting HIV, hepatitis C, and who knows what else. In places with both substance abuse treatment programs and needle exchange programs, they really work cooperatively on this issue.

---

4. On the relationship between access to sterile syringes, injecting behavior, and HIV risk, see Bluthenthal et al. 2007, Deren et al. 2006, Heimer et al. 1998, Heller et al. 2009, and Neaigus et al. 2008.

In the interests of protecting the public health, perhaps especially that of the so-called general population,[5] SEP advocates argue that the state has a responsibility to care for the health of the vulnerable and the addicted, who are otherwise unable to prevent their own HIV infection. It is IDUs' compromised will (Valverde 1998; Campbell 2007), the raging HIV epidemic, and the risk IDUs pose to the "general population" that bring IDUs to the attention of the state's public health agencies and that qualify them for the controversial benefits offered by SEPs. Addiction is translated into a demonstrable preexisting condition that paradoxically renders this marginalized population visible to the state, guaranteeing their eligibility for SEPs. For example, at another community meeting, Dr. Philip Weaver, architect of the CHA program described in Part I, spoke in his capacity as the medical director for a community health center that cares for many patients with AIDS. Weaver argued that the state had an obligation to provide care and treatment for active drug users. "So let's talk about substance abuse treatment," Dr. Weaver began. "I mean, seriously. We have wonderful treatment programs in the city that are dramatically underfunded." After explaining how outreach workers spend hours driving IDUs to residential drug treatment programs in far-flung places, he concluded. "We need to figure out how to get community control over the kinds of services we have here in [Thornton]." Marguerite, the coordinator of a local IDU drop-in center, chimed in, "The city needs to recognize that it has an obligation to its constituents."

The political novelty of this statement is Marguerite's insertion of active drug users into the body politic as constituents, a move countered by other local representatives who would place harm reduction and HIV prevention efforts squarely in the rhetorical and practical domain of law and order. For example, in an in-depth interview, city councilor Carlos Garcia lamented the politicization of Thornton's HIV prevention efforts. Drawing on an understanding of a "social contract" in which "the public ced[es] authority in matters of health to official expertise" (Horton and Barker 2009, 788), Garcia suggested that the Thornton Public Health Council would be better qualified to set public health policy than local politicians:

> I mean, we do have a public health council in [Thornton], and I believe that the public health council has come out in support of needle exchange, ah, and I think it probably should have been left at that. Again, I'm not sure that [*pauses*] there is a way at this point. In other communities that have passed the needle exchange, for example, it wasn't by politicians. Some people, you know, it's squarely within their hands, [and we need to] kind of take it out

5. See Waldby 1996 on the multiple politicized meanings of the term *general population* in AIDS discourse.

of their hands. I'm sure that politicians could do, you know, ah, be more than happy to give control of this issue, ah, so maybe it requires some kind of legislative change. I'm not sure.

Community members and politicians alike weigh the political and social implications of each position—appearing to "support drug users," like Mary Norris, the undecided city councilor, or ceding control to advocates or professional bodies such as the public health council, as Carlos Garcia recommends. Each of these moves reveals a broader set of views regarding the appropriate role of government, NGOs, and citizens, including local representatives' feelings about how they want themselves to be governed. If the state's syringe exchange law articulates IDUs as clients rather than criminals, they are entitled to publicly funded benefits such as sterile syringes but not health care, yet local representatives both adhere to and resist these constructions as they participate in state-mandated rituals of local approval. SEP advocates in Thornton felt that their best arguments for constructing IDUs as clients and beneficiaries lay in situating syringe exchange within a broader continuum of care, one with diverse effects on the subjectivities of those who enter into it.

Fetishization of Syringes

Advocates for syringe exchange frequently discuss the continuum of care as a counter to what they see as the public's fascination with syringes themselves as the principal element in SEPs. This fascination was articulated by Leo DiGiacomo, the director of WeCare, a Connecticut AIDS service organization, in a meeting with several Connecticut SEPs: "Because they just see it as needles, all they see is needles going back and forth. When in fact that's the *last* thing that happens in the interaction." Another participant at the meeting called for "changing the image of needle exchange to encourage support" among state legislators. Broadening the issue to focus on the continuum of care, DiGiacomo suggested, might provide supporters in the state legislature "political cover." Alan Dohan, another SEP advocate at the meeting, suggested bringing state legislators to the SEP vans that cover several Connecticut cities to "have them see what goes on, the breadth and depth of the interactions" between SEP staff and IDUs. Gary Johnson, another city councilor, addressed this question of public perceptions of syringe exchange in an in-depth interview with me as he pointed to the need for greater public understanding of the continuum of care:

People have this image that it's just handing out needles and that there's no personal contact. That's why I want to call it promoting clean needles rather than needle exchange. They just think of some junkies shootin' up in their backyard. They see it as a bad thing.

Instead, they have to see that people get full counseling, that they try to hook users into services by giving them something that they want, like syringes. Also they test for HIV. . . . You also have to educate the community on what needle exchange is like and have some leadership from *within* the community.

At a show-and-tell visit to the Highpoint SEP sponsored by Vanguard Health for members of the Thornton City Council, Highpoint director Chris Collins explained that the first goal of needle exchange is to have ongoing contact with the users. In her welcoming remarks opening the presentation, Waterford mayor Jennifer Jo Davis said, "It's unfortunate that the issue gets so politicized because this is really a public health issue. We're talking about addicts—I feel so much better about the fact that every time they come in here, it's an opportunity for them to talk with someone who will say to them, 'You don't have to live like this; we're here to help you.'"

Similarly, Maxine Washington, an outreach worker from Thornton, described her job as "building relationships, so that one day when someone is ready [to get into treatment], you're there." Speaking at a Thornton City Council meeting in favor of SEPs, Washington said that it might take months of giving people condoms and bleach kits, seeing people every week, until finally after three or four months someone would come to her and talk to her about getting into treatment. These kinds of personal relationships that are fostered in the context of a SEP seem to fill an important role for both SEP participants and staff. Staff understand their affective connections with participants as a significant part of IDUs' social networks, while participants may have few people in their lives with whom they can speak openly about their habit.

In offering IDUs sterile syringes to protect their health, SEPs do not decouple syringes from risk but instead heighten perceptions of syringe use as inherently risky by emphasizing the importance of always using a sterile syringe. By tying the provision of sterile syringes to the exchange of used syringes, SEPs continually affirm the ingrained, repetitive nature of addiction as well as its inescapability, at the same time as they attempt to link users with drug treatment services in pursuit of a cure (Small et al. 2010). Providing sterile syringes to IDUs only in exchange for used ones is itself a political compromise that sought to balance IDUs' need to inject with a sterile syringe every time (as recommended by the U.S. Centers for Disease Control) with the state's need to not appear to be "handing out syringes" and thereby supporting drug use. This view was paraphrased by an African American pastor who personally supported SEPs but described to me the arguments of those opposed:

So it's kind of like, "Well, you'll deal with the AIDS problem but not the drug problem." It makes us look as if we're choosing one evil over the other. "Well, we'll cut AIDS, but we'll let you all get high." You know. There's the argument "Well, if we're handing out drugs, if we're handing out needles, aren't we 'endorsing' drug use? Can't we find out where these guys are getting their drugs from and get the drug dealers and the users off the street?" Because drugs are a serious plague in our community, especially the African American community. So when you look at what drugs mean to some people, anything affiliated with it is evil: the user, the needle, and the supplier. So how dare we supply any one of those things? It's kind of as if we're giving a stamp of endorsement on it.

In other words, IDUs qualify for state assistance in the form of sterile syringes only *insofar as* they are already in the abject position of drug users and maintain that position by actively using syringes in order to obtain new ones.

Governance of Syringe Exchange Programs

SEPs emerged as specific technologies grown from harm reduction movements that existed before the HIV epidemic but received an enormous increase in attention and support with the advent of the HIV epidemic among IDUs (Inciardi and Harrison 2000; Roe 2005).[6] While syringe exchange is often touted as a highly cost-effective HIV prevention method, Ricky Bluthenthal (1998) argues that SEPs have not emerged "through the rational . . . application of the most promising and cost effective strategies as understood by public health experts" but, rather, "through the mobilization of [affected] communities and their allies" demanding resources to address the raging HIV epidemic in their communities (1998, 1151). Bluthenthal emphasizes that SEPs were implemented as a result of grassroots activism and policy advocacy *in advance of* the widespread dissemination of scientific evidence of SEP effectiveness in preventing HIV. Later, with the advent of AIDS, SEPs and their sponsoring organizations began to demand state support for their efforts that was on a par with resources invested in other publicly supported HIV prevention measures such as health education or condom distribution campaigns. In and around Thornton, several community organizations used the SEP issue (embedded as it was in broader discussions around HIV, drug use, and marginalization) as a field in which they were able to stake claims and take positions in relation to the larger body politic (Shaw 2006). Thus syringe exchange

---

6. For instance, the director of Vanguard Health Systems, which runs the Waterford SEP, reported in an interview that "we [Vanguard] had dealt with some issues related to addiction, but the way that we came to [run an SEP] was really through the issue of AIDS, not through the issue of addiction."

emerged as a form of grassroots organizing that later became more closely articulated with state practices of HIV prevention (Geary 2007) as some programs obtained state funding and sought to enlist IDUs in practicing and propagating harm reduction norms.

SEPs try to manage the contradictory demands placed on them (to provide sterile syringes to IDUs along with referrals to other kinds of services, and to protect the health of the general population) through a variety of policies and procedures. As SEPs become increasingly institutionalized, like the outreach worker programs portrayed in Part I, new forms of accountability may be imposed on them. For example, techniques for tracking syringes circulated by SEPs evolved in part in response to criticisms of the state's role in providing tools for illicit behavior as well as legislators' and others' articulated fears that SEPs pose a risk to the "general population." SEPs are governed by the requirements and constraints associated with public funding and legislation that may authorize, forbid, or ignore the existence of such programs. Varying state mandates govern SEP workers as well as the IDUs who attend state programs.

To explore the difference that state support or lack thereof makes in the actual practices of SEPs, researchers tracked changes in SEP performance in California between 2000 and 2002, following passage of that state's local approval law (Bluthenthal et al. 2008).[7] Some analysts have expressed concern that state recognition and funding comes at the price of increased surveillance over and greater restrictions on syringe exchange procedures; in contrast, Bluthenthal and colleagues found that "approved programs, compared with unapproved programs, did not become more restrictive in their dispensation policies [and further] reported fewer syringe and supply shortages." Approved programs also had bigger budgets than unapproved programs (Bluthenthal et al. 2008, 281).

Other reviews have identified constraints associated with state sponsorship that may negatively impact SEP effectiveness, especially on those who

---

7. AB136, passed by the California legislature in 2000, forbids prosecution of any "public entity, its agents, or employees . . . for distribution of hypodermic needles or syringes to participants in clean needle and syringe exchange projects authorized by the public entity pursuant to a declaration of a local emergency due to the existence of a critical local public health crisis" (qtd. in Bluthenthal et al. 2008, 278). Before this, the so-called emergency defense had been successfully used to defend syringe exchange workers in court (the emergency defense argued that civil disobedience—breaking the law against distributing syringes without a prescription—was required by the public health emergency of the HIV epidemic). As in Massachusetts, the California law does not specifically sanction syringe exchange but creates the possibility of "local approval," here couched in terms of a public health emergency. Note that syringe recipients are identified in the text of the law as "participants" rather than drug users, already signaling their relationship to the state as clients rather than criminals. Note as well that the state of exception being constructed here, *contra* Agamben, suspends the usual state business of prosecution in favor, instead, of potentially life-saving technologies of syringe exchange.

do not directly use the program themselves. For example, a small number of IDUs in Thornton saved their own and others' used syringes to periodically exchange at the Waterford SEP. They might pool their resources for a bus ticket or pay a friend to drive them twenty miles up the highway to the Highpoint program, where they would receive dozens or even hundreds of sterile syringes in return and continue to exchange these sterile syringes for their friends and contacts in Thornton. This process, called secondary or satellite exchange (Valente et al. 1998), is an important way for SEPs to extend the reach of their networks of exchange (Lorvick et al. 2006). In a review article on SEP effectiveness in preventing HIV infection, Francisco Bastos and Steffanie Strathdee observed:

> In Baltimore, satellite exchangers comprised only 10% of SEP attenders, but accounted for 64% of all needles distributed (Valente et al. 1998). Examples of IDUs who may be reached through satellite exchange are persons who are secretly injecting (e.g. IDUs on parole, in prison, hospital or drug treatment programmes), shooting gallery attenders, persons who do not perceive themselves as IDUs (e.g. steroid injectors . . .) and IDUs who do not live in an area served by a SEP. (2000, 1773)

Bastos and Strathdee identify "local contextual factors" in SEP effectiveness that include funding restrictions, legal recognition, and other resources. They comment:

> Strict one-for-one exchange policies are often required by policy makers to placate concerns that SEPs could encourage initiation of injection among youth. . . . In an attempt to achieve a "high access" rather than a "high volume" model that focuses on direct contact with each IDU, some SEPs have actively discouraged secondary exchange, a practice which could limit SEP effectiveness since coverage [the availability of sterile syringes in a given area] is reduced. (2000, 1774)

These authors point to the hazards associated with the strict enforcement of 1:1 exchange policies engendered by concerns around political liability (see also Bluthenthal et al. 2007; Heller et al. 2009). Dr. Robert Heimer, a researcher at the Yale University Department of Epidemiology and Public Health and co-investigator on the Syringe Access project discussed in Chapter 5, proposed eliminating Connecticut's 1:1 cap on syringe exchange, arguing that the "ideal system is to ask people how many syringes they need for themselves and people they're providing care for [i.e., secondary exchangers] and give it to them." Heimer further "stated that a worker on a van cannot tell an active IDU what they need, but they can tell them how to protect themselves and provide clients with the tools" to do so.[8] These policies impose their own regimes of accountability on the practice of syringe exchange, as illustrated in media representations of SEPs:

> It's needle exchange day at the Luis Llorens Torres housing project and throughout Puerto Rico's capital city. Members of the Community Initiative, the island's only needle-exchange group, have set out buckets for addicts to drop their used needles into as the workers count out clean ones. "Thirty-one, thirty-two, thirty-three," says one woman, as she drops her used needles into a bucket beneath a large tree. Those who show up receive exactly the number of needles they hand over. (Collie 2001, 1A)

This excerpt shows the active participation of users in these regimes of accountability, as the woman quoted is reciting aloud the number of syringes she returns.

Such practices of accountability interact in complex and sometimes arcane ways with techniques of identification and anonymity. For example, on a visit to the Highpoint program in May 2004, Thornton city councilor Gary Johnson asked how people are identified when they come into the exchange. Chris Collins, the Highpoint director, explained that the state requires that while users must be enrolled members of a SEP, the exchange itself must be anonymous (i.e., no names are used in the accounting of each individual exchange). The membership card has a unique personal identifier on it so that Highpoint can track how many syringes a person exchanges and what services they receive. When a new user walks into the office, Collins said, SEP staff get her interested in the program, register her, create a membership card, do the exchange, offer prevention and safety information, and provide her with referrals such as to treatment programs. In response to the visitors' concerns that the increasing number of syringes in local circulation might somehow harm the "general population," Collins reported that about 90 percent of the syringes they gave out came back to the program. While a secondary exchanger in Thornton who used this program later told me that bulk exchangers seldom actually count the syringes they return but instead estimate to the nearest hundred, those in the audience for this discussion with Collins seemed reassured by the idea that someone is keeping track of how many syringes come into and go out of the program.

Collins explained that Highpoint operates under a 1:1+1 policy: users who return one syringe can get two back. The program developed this rule after turning away an IDU who came to the program asking for a

---

8. This is as reported in the Connecticut HIV Community Planning Group newsletter, January 6, 2003. Observe how Heimer lapses into the individualizing "protect yourself" language of harm reduction discussed in the previous chapter.

syringe when it operated under a strict 1:1 policy, but he did not bring a used one to exchange. The idea of a "starter kit" that includes a sterile syringe provided to a person on his first visit who did not offer the SEP a used syringe in exchange proved to be quite controversial when it spread in the course of Thornton's debates about syringe exchange. The controversy centered on fears that the "starter kit" would, as cited by Francisco Bastos and Steffanie Strathdee previously, entice users to switch to injecting from other methods of use such as snorting or even to initiate drug use altogether.[9] Collins defended the 1:1+1 policy by reiterating the program's desire to establish an ongoing relationship with IDUs, saying, "If you turn them away empty-handed, they won't come back."[10] Similarly, at a community forum I attended on syringe exchange in Thornton in March 2004, Jerome Richardson, an African American SEP supporter who worked for an AIDS service organization that publicly and prominently opposed SEPs, spoke of systems of "accountability" like labeled syringes, so that people in the community could tell if the syringes from the SEP were being discarded or returned. "I'm not asking for a one hundred percent return rate," he said, "but if we could show that even *most* of them were being returned," he thought that would help. Though he supports needle exchange, he commented that "we give the opposition a lot of material" to use when SEP advocates fail to include detailed regimes of accountability in calls for syringe exchange for Thornton's IDUs. "You got to take away the opposition's ammunition; that's the only way to get [SEPs in Thornton]," Richardson concluded. Regimes of accountability are here proposed as a means of both strategically eliminating opponents' "ammunition" and as a means of governing SEPs themselves.

Other SEPs, however, prefer elements of illegality (operating in defiance of state laws banning the sale or distribution of hypodermic syringes). At the 2002 conference of the North American Syringe Exchange Network (NASEN) in Albuquerque, New Mexico, for instance, I observed an informal plenary session where syringe exchange workers shared their experiences with these and other mechanisms of accountability. The panel organizers distinguished among several degrees of legality for SEPs ranging from "underground" (illegal and operating below the radar of law enforcement recognition or surveillance) to "tolerated" (referring to programs that were not technically legal but were implicitly allowed by law enforcement to exist) to state-funded (as in four localities in Massachusetts). Interestingly, some syringe exchange workers attending the plenary seemed to long for

---

9. Harm reduction advocates dismiss these fears as ludicrous, yet their persuasive power is indicated by their continued circulation across sites (e.g., Baltimore, Montreal, Thornton) and over time.

10. Despite this observation, in thirty-five SEPs surveyed by Bluthenthal and colleagues (2008), 1:1 exchange was the most common exchange policy (practiced by 33 percent of programs).

the discretion and freedom that was partly enabled by underground status. According to these speakers, illegality, operating with entirely donated funds and supplies, implied much less paperwork, less accountability with both funding and syringes, and no need for ID cards. On the other hand, participants at this meeting echoed the findings reported earlier by Bluthenthal and colleagues (2008) as they complained about a constant shortage of supplies, as well as the ever-present risk of arrest and frequent burnout among volunteer or underpaid staff members. SEPs in the United States operate in a sociopolitical landscape patterned by a range of local, state, and federal laws that authorize, prohibit, or remain silent on their existence. The following section briefly outlines some features and consequences of ambivalent state support for syringe exchange in Massachusetts before turning to the ways in which these conditions contour the governing mentalities of SEPs as they interact with IDUs in practice.

Ambivalent State Support for Syringe Exchange

As they participate in collective struggles over the best way to ensure the public health, states alternately support and disavow syringe exchange as an HIV prevention technology.[11] Massachusetts authorized the first pilot SEP in July 1993, with the stipulation that it be "implemented and regulated by the Department of Public Health [DPH] with local cooperation" (Young and Wunsch 2002). The legislators' failure to specify what exactly constituted "local cooperation," however, led to struggles within localities over which governmental bodies were qualified to give local approval. Boston and Cambridge jointly operated the first pilot program without incident after obtaining approval from both city councils. Two years later, the legislature amended the 1993 law to allow ten DPH-sponsored SEPs. By 1995, programs were operating in two more Massachusetts towns.

The state law explicitly makes this health policy decision a question of and for local government.[12] In Waterford, "local cooperation" was

---

11. At the 2002 NASEN plenary session mentioned earlier, for example, someone from a state health department said that his health department was legally prohibited from running a syringe exchange itself but that he had several hundred thousand dollars and thirty thousand syringes that he would like to give to an AIDS service organization or another community-based organization to operate an exchange. None of the organizations he had approached were willing to take on the task because its legality in that state was questionable, however. Other participants in the plenary suggested that the speaker encourage a community-based organization to create programs for active users to both establish relationships with that population and to create a plausible "smokescreen" under which the organization might operate an SEP. In this instance, an actual agent of the state was actively involved in encouraging others to (possibly) circumvent the laws of that state for the purpose of preventing HIV among IDUs.

12. In a paper analyzing the effects of local approval laws compared with statewide support, Ricky Bluthenthal and colleagues observe, "Statewide funding and implementation

implemented with support from the mayor and police chief, at the request of the Vanguard Health Systems HIV prevention unit. Chris Collins, Highpoint's director, recalls, "The mayor . . . agreed to support [SEPs in Waterford] as long as we could get the chief of police on board, and we didn't talk about it till after the election, and that's what we did." The Massachusetts legislature took a similar tack on the question of whether schools could distribute condoms to high school students. Torn between the progressive desire to give young people the tools to protect themselves from sexually transmitted infections and the fear that doing so would leave legislators vulnerable to conservative charges of "endorsing" teen sexual activity, the legislature tossed the question to local school boards while giving overall permission for condom distribution in high schools. In an in-depth interview with me in 2004, Candace Cartwright, the executive director of Vanguard Health Systems (which runs the Highpoint program), commented:

> I really do see real parallels with the condom distribution issue. In Massachusetts, . . . instead of allowing high schools to have condoms, what the legislature did was to say that locales needed to vote to decide whether a high school could have condoms. And so there were terrible fights, school boards who voted, [and] very progressive people who were on school boards were voted out. And so, with that experience, it was kind of like, "Let's be careful about needle exchange." So I was actually involved in helping to craft the law that allowed the demonstration [needle exchange] projects to happen, and it was a real compromise. I was very sorry for the local option, but again at that point, it was all—it was the best that we could do, and I don't think anyone thought it was gonna be such a hard fight.

The "hard fight" Cartwright refers to was the 1998 referendum in Thornton that defeated SEPs by a margin of 10 percent, organized by a group of local activists opposed to SEPs. The referendum followed a vote in favor of SEPs by the Thornton City Council in March 1998; after the referendum, the city council reversed itself in another vote and has stood in opposition to SEPs ever since.[13]

---

appear most effective in obtaining rapid and comprehensive deployment of [syringe exchange]. Local-approval approaches have been unsuccessful in other states (Massachusetts, Ohio, and Pennsylvania) and our study found mixed results in California" (Bluthenthal et al. 2008, 282).

13. SEP advocates continued to lobby the city council for SEP in Thornton from 1998 until 2006, as recounted in part here, when Massachusetts decriminalized the sale of hypodermic needles in June 2006, following more than forty states in allowing syringes to be purchased without a doctor's prescription.

The successful intervention of organizations such as Vanguard Health Systems in implementing an HIV prevention program for IDUs demonstrates one way in which the state as an agent of governing is now relocated "as simply one element . . . in multiple circuits of power, connecting a diversity of authorities and forces, within a whole variety of complex assemblages" (Rose 1999, 5). As state-supported programs primarily run by private nonprofit organizations, SEPs exemplify the concept of assemblage outlined by Rose (1999).[14] Marguerite, the drop-in center coordinator quoted previously, described her vision of the role of SEPs in this larger assemblage: "[We had wanted to make] needle exchange a referral funnel, a potential referral tunnel, and that was another way of guaranteeing that folks would get access to care. At this point, it's still being proposed as a very underfunded program. [But] the whole perspective about needle exchange being part of the continuum of care is much more acceptable now." The continuum of care described by Marguerite came into existence in part as a result of state legislators' desire to protect the public health while avoiding controversy and displacing responsibility onto the local level. Unique local assemblages of nonprofit organizations and local police forces were submerged into larger networks when Massachusetts replaced program-specific ID cards with a single statewide membership card to emphasize the state's endorsement of SEPs *across* localities. Chris Collins, director of the Highpoint program, complained.

> Chris: Well, I had some issues with [the state card, in terms of losing] the unique identity of the different programs. . . . Like in the [Waterford] program, the telephone number of the [Waterford] Police Department was on [our ID card], and that was going to be lost when we went to a state[wide] card. And that was a big thing; that was something [the police chief] wanted so that he could connect with other police officers that had questions, and that would have been lost. And the more the focus is on statewide, and so, just kind of like invisibility, I think. [*Laughs.*] Just kind of wanting to promote the [Waterford] program too. It had a number of issues. And eventually I was able to let go of it, but it took a while. The [state AIDS agency's] perspective was that it would help to reinforce the fact that this was a statewide program and that you register in one city but it's good for wherever. And so that's what they eventually did. Three months

14. Nikolas Rose (1999) rearticulates Gilles Deleuze and Felix Guattari's concept of assemblage (1987). While Deleuze and Guattari emphasize the machinic aspects of an assemblage as well as its operation as desire, building on psychoanalytic theory, Rose places this concept firmly in the domain of neoliberal governance. My use of the term here is closer to Rose's formulation than Deleuze and Guattari's.

ago we switched to that, and so we stopped using our own cards. The new blue card, it's very pretty. Have you seen them?
Susan: I need to get one. I have that old yellow card.
Chris: And it has the state logo on it, so it looks very official. So it's a good thing.

Following a court case (*Commonwealth v. Landry*, 2002) in which a member of the Cambridge SEP was charged with possession of illegal syringes while she was arrested on a shoplifting charge in a neighboring town, Massachusetts switched to a single statewide SEP membership ID.[15] The new ID, a thoroughly biopolitical technology, was designed to improve the efficiency of the continuum of care at the same time that it conflicted with the aims of "grassroots" harm reduction programs as they coupled with local police forces and state public health agencies.

The ambivalence revealed by this case as well as by city councilors I interviewed who struggled with balancing law-and-order interpretations of drug use with public health mandates played out in complex ways. Similar to the ways in which SEPs in many states grapple with police harassment of both IDUs and SEP staff (Singer, Weeks, and Himmelgreen 1995; Heimer et al. 1996; Bluthenthal 1998), SEPs themselves enact conflicting tendencies toward empowerment and constraint as they provide syringes to IDUs to prevent HIV infections.

The Governing Mentalities of Programs for Drug Users

As state-supported programs aimed at reducing HIV infection and funneling drug users into services, Massachusetts SEPs sought to foster particular forms of subjectivity among IDUs. Linking users with drug treatment programs and facilitating their admission thereto is another way the state is able to manage the problematic population of illicit drug users. As discussed in the previous chapter, harm reduction, in emphasizing the personal behaviors drug users ought to follow to protect their own and

---

15. Maria Landry showed the arresting officers her SEP card and informed them that she was permitted to carry the sterile syringes, but the police proceeded with the arrest and charges. The Massachusetts Supreme Judicial Court found that membership in any state-approved SEP allowed one to carry sterile syringes anywhere in the state and, further, to exchange syringes at any state-sponsored program. In this case, two arms of the state were working at cross purposes, as law enforcement sought to hold Maria Landry accountable to its interpretation of legal code banning the possession of sterile syringes without a doctor's prescription, while the public health department sought to allow SEP members to obtain and carry sterile syringes anywhere in the state to encourage harm reduction practices among IDUs. See also Akhil Gupta and Aradhana Sharma on the "everyday material objects . . . that bear the stamp, seal or signature of the state [that] also help to construct and represent 'the state'" (2006, 279), located here as a force authorizing the assemblage of actors, institutions, and objects that is syringe exchange.

others' health, espouses the self-regulation of drug users in its emphasis on "controlled use" rather than complete abstinence (e.g., Duff 2004). While participation in a SEP lowers one's risk for HIV seroconversion, drug user conduct remains an issue in local debates over syringe exchange.[16] SEPs govern the conduct of drug users as they regulate the number of syringes that IDUs may receive and the conditions under which they may do so, "compel[ling] addicts to have multiple points of contact with professionals where the virtues of treatment and detox are impressed on them" (Small et al. 2010).

SEPs, especially state-funded programs, are accountable to diverse political ends and public health goals, including but not limited to reducing HIV rates among IDUs, reducing the numbers of discarded syringes in public areas, and increasing the numbers of IDUs who enter drug treatment programs. SEPs also enact their own forms of accountability on the IDUs who attend, assigning them anonymous or individual IDs and tracking the number of syringes they exchange as well as the number and types of HIV risk behaviors they engage in. "This dependence of regimes of practices on forms of knowledge accounts for [their] associat[ion] with . . . definite, explicit *programmes*, i.e., deliberate and relatively systematic forms of thought that endeavor to transform those practices" (Dean 1999, 22). And yet, while SEPs, state departments of public health, and harm reduction organizations each aim to transform the practices as well as the subjectivities of IDUs, these regimes of practice routinely fail to regulate IDUs' behavior: for instance, IDUs do not always adhere to harm reduction recommendations to use a sterile syringe for every injection (Heller et al. 2009). Thornton IDUs are seldom able to travel to the nearest SEP, twenty miles away in Waterford. Some secondary exchangers in Thornton who attend the Highpoint program collect their friends' syringes, then exchange and return them, while others sold the Highpoint syringes to Thornton users for five dollars apiece (an exorbitant price at a time when a bag of heroin was selling for ten dollars, or a bundle—ten bags—for fifty dollars). As SEPs govern IDUs through services, states seek to discharge their responsibilities to promote the public health by outsourcing those tasks to

---

16. Dozens of epidemiological studies have demonstrated SEPs to be effective in reducing the rate of HIV infection among IDUs (Bastos and Strathdee 2000; Buchanan et al. 2004; Des Jarlais et al. 2009). Ethnographic studies (sociological, anthropological, and public health) of syringe exchange have been completed by Bluthenthal (1998); Broadhead et al. (1999); Hagan, Des Jarlais, and Purchase (1993); and Singer, Romero-Daza, et al. (1995), among others. These studies emphasize themes similar to those explored here but typically (with the exception of Bastos and Strathdee 2000 and Heimer et al. 1996) focus more on program participants rather than staff. This chapter focuses on SEP staff because of their uniquely situated perspectives as both former IDUs themselves (often) and as agents of programs that govern participants through providing them services. At the same time, SEP staff are fettered by the demands of state and other funding through the regimes of accountability explored here.

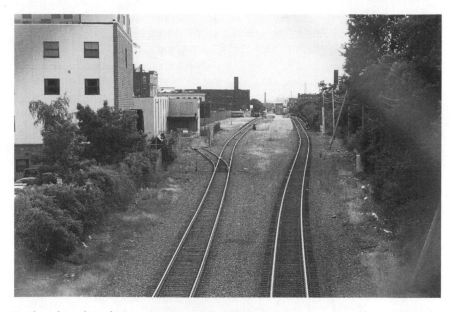

Railroad tracks, often overgrown with shrubbery, provide an out-of-the-way gathering place for Thornton's injection drug users. *(Photograph courtesy of Amanda Quinby.)*

harm reduction organizations often staffed by people who are themselves in recovery from addiction. Following the same governing mentality of "like helping like" portrayed in Chapter 2, state lawmakers and public health administrators deem harm reduction organizations as best suited to offer syringe exchange and other services to IDUs, who hover at the margins of the body politic. IDUs most likely to use such programs, meanwhile, are caught within constraints imposed by conditions of poverty and advanced marginalization (Feldman 2001).

From a user's perspective, syringe exchange addresses the problem of having to pay for syringes sold by diabetics, drug users, or syringe-selling middlemen. One former IDU described using a syringe exchange when he lived in New Haven, Connecticut: "It was great. It was good to be able to not have to look around or, you know, do all kinds of stuff—drive crazy places to buy a syringe from a diabetic somewhere . . . or you just ask the friend that was with you and I didn't think [whether] they were sick or not, just gimme some water."[17] When I asked outreach workers and SEP advocates, many of whom are themselves people in recovery from drug

17. Observe the shift from second to first person at the end of this quote as the speaker inserts himself into the subjective judgment "I didn't think [whether] they were sick *or not*"–indicating a moment of post hoc consideration of risk that did not occur as the desire for a fix overcame him—"just gimme some water" with which he will perhaps rinse the syringe that his friend, sick or not, has just used to inject himself.

addiction, why Thornton should have an SEP, they described drug users' failure to adhere to recommended HIV prevention behaviors: "They go, 'It's clean; it's clean!' [If I ask,] 'Well, you don't use the bleach?' [They say,] 'No, I don't use no bleach; I don't need no bleach.' And then you got to go through the education once again and explain, but they don't wanna hear that. 'I'm in a hurry; I gotta hurry up, so what you wanna tell me?' And sometimes they don't use the bleach. Some of them use it, but the majority, they don't want to use it." Or, as another former-user-turned-outreach-worker described, "We'd pick up syringes off the damn floor and clean them. . . . I don't know how I didn't [*knocks on wood*]—I didn't get sick. You know, because I shoot up with some people that were sick [had AIDS]." A participant in the Syringe Access study explained, "When you're [drug-]sick, you don't think them things. You just think you want to use."[18]

The micropractices of drug use these former addicts describe are shaped by economic conditions of access to prevention tools such as bleach, running water, and shelter from the scanning eyes of police officers, as well as the political conditions that determine the availability of SEPs or pharmacy access to sterile syringes (Buchanan et al. 2002). All these circumstances make up the habitus of drug use that is the target of harm reduction interventions. In an article on the use of prescription heroin as a substitute for methadone, Philippe Bourgois presents field notes from a visit to a Swiss supervised injection site that illuminate the intimate, repetitive nature of injection practice. Bourgois observes, "The nurse walks over to the tattooed man [and says], 'Are you ready yet for me to administer you the injection?' She looks up at me [Bourgois] to explain, 'We try to break them of the habit of their gestures by administering the injections for them.' He nods meekly and allows her to complete the injection for him. He then turns to me and talks about how much 'progress' he is making by disassociating himself from the gesture of injecting" (2002, 264). A great deal of effort has been invested in spreading the harm reduction norms "Don't share your works" and "Always clean your needles," because for people who have been injecting drugs for years, if not decades, the act of injecting itself (what Bourgois translates as "the habit of their gestures") becomes highly routinized and individual to each drug user. As a prelude to "the fix," the intense gratification of the first moment of a drug rush, the gestures of injecting are invested with enormous personal significance

18. Addiction to heroin can be identified by withdrawal symptoms that come on surprisingly few hours after one's last use. As explained by Parker, the white SEP worker at Highpoint quoted previously, many people do not realize that with habitual use (urban lore has it, as few as three days in a row), heroin use is characterized less by the experience of euphoria and more by the abatement of withdrawal symptoms, which can include nausea, diarrhea, weakness, tremors, and runny nose. Long-term heroin users thus would describe using heroin to me as "getting well" rather than getting high. Withdrawal is also known as drug-sickness.

and may thus prove resistant to outside modification. SEPs are envisioned as a structural intervention to increase the availability of syringes in a given community and thus decrease the risk of HIV infection posed by any single syringe (Heimer et al. 1998); by embedding the act of exchange syringes within a broader continuum of care and providing referrals to drug treatment programs, SEPs also work to manage the behavior of IDUs in an effort to promote their, and the public's, health.

SEPs and the Continuum of Care

Ethnically and economically marginalized drug users in Thornton, and elsewhere, are not unfamiliar with the complex web of social services that shape their access to food, housing, income, health care, and education. As explored in Part I, health care and housing agencies in Thornton are typically experienced as holding determinative power and authority over the lives of those seeking aid from them; by offering "wrap-around" services, SEPs (especially those offered by health departments or AIDS service agencies) risk locating themselves among these service providers viewed by IDUs as requiring some kind of tribute (not only used syringes, but information about their health, risk behaviors, or sexual orientation) in order to receive "free" sterile syringes.[19] Many SEPs present themselves as the product of grassroots organizing by drug users (often, former addicts) for drug users specifically to combat this attitude among clients (Bluthenthal 1998). Nonetheless, as Aradhana Sharma (2008) and others have shown, the provision of services, even empowerment-based services, is an important way of managing and reforming the conduct of marginalized and stigmatized populations. As explored in the previous chapter, enlisting drug users' participation in and commitment to the aims of harm reduction, for example, and inculcating an attitude of "prevention" among habitual users are elements in the construction of new subjectivities shaped as much by neoliberal imperatives as by histories of drug user organizing for better health.

At a meeting of the public safety committee of the Thornton City Council, several speakers pointed out the need for education to be a critical part of a proposed SEP, which attendees seemed to agree would work best as a mobile service. Leshawna Bailey, a former drug user who now worked

---

19. Some SEPs extend this ethic of care even further and offer coffee, food, or personal hygiene items to users who stop by the syringe exchange van or office. One argument in favor of "wraparound services" offered by SEPs is the destigmatization of the site itself: if people have many different kinds of reasons to visit an SEP, including free condoms, HIV testing, or foodstuffs, others may be less likely to identify the visitor as an IDU. See also Ben Peacock (2008), who explores in greater detail the increasing inter-implication of service and research, especially around marginalized populations and AIDS prevention services.

as a secondary exchanger in Thornton, emphasized that needles should not be the only thing on the van. Everyone who worked there would be trained to offer referrals to other agencies to link people with drug treatment, food stamps, housing, and health care. City councilor Marisa Ruccione asked Bailey, "And what if they say, 'No, no, no'?" Several SEP advocates acknowledged that would happen occasionally, arguing that councilors should think of the SEP van as triage; as Dr. Weaver put it, "you can't do surgery in a [van]—all you can do is assess people for what they need, and then send them elsewhere to get it." Denise Murphy, the public health commissioner, stood up in the audience and said that giving a sterile syringe even to a user who does not want any other services is still reducing the harm to the community.

SEP advocates argued against stigmatizing constructions of drug users by seeking to humanize users and emphasizing the social relationships between SEP staff and participants. For instance, at a 2004 community meeting on needle exchange in Williamsburg, a predominantly African American neighborhood of Thornton, Frank Stein argued:

> Once you have a habit, heroin addicts don't like being addicted to heroin. No one wants to stay a junkie, just like no one wants to be poor. It sucks. People want to get their lives together, but they need help. That's what a needle exchange offers, a place where people talk to you. "How you doing today?" "Not so great, man. I'm sick of this. I really want to quit." "Great. We can hook you up with a program." "I don't know. I don't know if I'm ready, though." "Okay. Whenever you're ready, we're here for you." Needle exchange keeps people alive so that people have a choice. What needle exchange offers is a continuum of care. The thing about HIV is drug treatment might get people sober, but then they die of AIDS, sober. It's happened to my friends. Statistics don't show what it feels like; that's why we get so frustrated with statistics. City councilors don't read them. It's the continuum of care that's important. [Thornton] needs to take the moral high ground and say, "We will support this as a means of reducing drug-related harm in [Thornton]."

Stein emphasized the social and temporal location of syringe exchange within the broader continuum of care as an institutional elaboration of the social relations that thus serve to humanize IDUs. Similarly, an active user I interviewed described the potential he saw in the continuum of care offered by SEPs, at the same time that he identified the syringe as the primary "object they desire":

> [I think they should] just provide the service [SEP], because at least if people are going to choose to do that, they can do it in a healthy

manner and possibly cut down on infectious diseases and provide education at the same time. Because they're going there to get the objects that they desire, a set of works. And while they're there, maybe someone can get through to them, or they'll see something and read about it and learn something. You know, it's not just one thing. Possibly more can come out of it. Or possibly they'll hear something, or someone will be able to empathize with them in such a manner that maybe they'll get help. Or maybe their life will become something that has a positive contribution to the community.

Here as well, the potential relationship between SEP staff member and IDU is an important feature of the continuum of care. By placing IDUs in relation to others, even paid staffers, SEP advocates and users work against widespread constructions of addicts as isolated and less than human in their dependence on illicit substances.

SEPs' manifest difficulty of achieving the Massachusetts mandate to link IDUs to treatment programs brings to light the role of SEPs as a technology of governing that is designed to fail. This was stated plainly in a meeting of the public safety committee of the Thornton City Council by a city councilor who had worked for decades as a parole officer, who observed, "Let's face it, the state is not interested in working with people on the street. They have made that very clear. I've never seen it so bad as it is now. There are no treatment beds, you can't get people treatment." If state legislators did not intend to fund more drug treatment beds to expand access and meet their mandate that SEPs link users to treatment programs, what were the "contradictory, messy, and refractory effects" (Li 2005, 391, citing Ferguson 1994) of this particular scheme to improve the human condition that seems doomed to failure? Relocating responsibility for health policy decisions such as HIV prevention to the local level creates further opportunities for "compromise and collusion" (Li 2005) between legislators and their voters. Yet the continuum of care in theory leading to drug treatment featured prominently in arguments made in favor of syringe exchange for Thornton.

Conclusion

As private nonprofit organizations operating with state funding, SEPs occupy a paradoxical space as part of a larger assemblage that acts on IDUs' conduct by engaging them in a continuum of care, supporting their drug use (by requiring the return of used syringes in order to obtain sterile ones), and facilitating their return to independence from drugs by entering them into drug treatment programs. This chapter aims to broaden the range of institutions we understand as governing bodies to include not just

NGOs but specifically organizations claiming to represent marginalized populations such as IDUs. The alignments forged among these institutions and the IDUs who use, staff, and administer them are unstable, conflicting, and subject to negotiation as different kinds of political actors contest interpretations of drug use and risk.

SEPs seem to provoke an especially thorny dilemma for legislators who worry that embracing a public health response to drug use instead of a criminal justice response will lead to a crisis of legitimacy with their supporters. They fear that a state policy of harm reduction and syringe exchange imperils their position as state representatives concerned with maintaining law and order. As explored in previous chapters, the rationalities of neoliberal governance take a distinctly *moral* form as ideologies of personal responsibility are embraced by, or imposed on, government activities and programs. Public disagreement over how to interpret and operationalize the ethical basis of government animates continuing debates over SEPs to prevent HIV infection among IDUs, who are placed at increased risk for HIV infection by structural factors largely beyond their control. In addition, while IDUs are generally *not* regarded as constituents (Shaw 2006) or as members of the body politic (Waldby 1996), SEPs in particular and harm reduction approaches more generally have emerged through their proactive political and community organizing.

As archetypes of what Aihwa Ong refers to as "excluded humanity" (2006, 24), IDUs are banished from the body politic because of their illicit drug use. In their addiction and abject dependence on illegal substances, IDUs paradigmatically fail to adhere to norms of independence and self-sufficiency that typify neoliberal U.S. ideals of citizenship. Paradoxically, however, their addiction and resulting risk for HIV infection also merit state support, contributing to a stigmatized kind of biocitizenship echoing that described by Adriana Petryna (2002) and João Biehl (2004).

Further, if, as Nikolas Rose and Carlos Novas suggest, "citizenship . . . is manifested in a range of struggles over individual identities, forms of collectivization, demands for recognition, access to knowledge, and claims to expertise" (2005, 442, citing Heath, Rapp, and Taussig 2004), current and former IDUs organizing around HIV prevention are engaged in expressions of citizenship at a more fundamental level. Like minority advocacy organizations who use health disparities to contest social inequality, IDUs and SEP advocates alike strive to transform social relations and structures of inequality by creating new institutions designed to bring their interests to the public sphere. South African anthropologist Steven Robins (2009) shows how the original humanitarian "bare life" concerns of AIDS treatment activists were broadened through coalition work with a "much broader political project aimed at addressing the daily conditions of poor people's lives" (638) that crystallized in the collective response to a sudden rise in xenophobic violence in South African townships in May 2008 (645).

Activists' broader focus in this South African case are likewise reflected in Thornton SEP advocates' efforts to embed calls for syringe exchange in a larger continuum of care.

As communities use debates about health care to define who does and does not belong to "the public" and who counts as a citizen, conceptions of entitlement work through and against these new constructions of difference as they designate the conditions and ailments that allow marginalized citizens access to additional resources. The continuum of care depends on users embracing the position of responsible addict (continuing to use syringes but returning their syringes to exchange for sterile ones, to be used for every injection) or the addict in recovery, if they enroll in drug treatment programs proffered through the continuum of care. A range of accountability mechanisms help construct and enforce new, responsibilized subject-positions for both IDUs and the people in recovery who frequently staff them. Conceived originally as grassroots organizations supporting drug users and resisting dominant norms of acceptable behavior and conduct, harm reduction organizations that sponsor SEPs struggle with new norms of responsibility and accountability to the state and other funders. As they work to maintain commitments to alternative views of drug use, and new configurations of society and entitlements, people in recovery, SEP staff and advocates provoke an ongoing reconsideration of what it means not only to be entitled but to be a citizen.

Conclusion

After college, I spent some time as an activist with the AIDS and women's health movements in New York City. I remember attending endless strategy sessions in advance of protest actions, trying to come up with our demands. (Never do an action without presenting demands!) In these conversations someone would often share this bit of social movement wisdom: when negotiating with the people in charge, ask for everything, because it increases the chances of getting what is most crucial. As I now observe diverse groups engaged in community health advocacy, it occurs to me that they may be practicing some version of this wisdom as they take up the banner of health in order to talk about inequality in the United States. Perhaps the activists, researchers, and advocates who call for remedies to health disparities that include social goods such as housing and health insurance are "asking for everything" in the hopes that what is most immediately needed in the short term—more Spanish-speaking medical interpreters in the hospital, for example—will be granted as a goodwill gesture in the absence of real structural reforms.

Anthropologists and others analyzing these moves can interpret the gains and deferrals that result from a strategy of "asking for everything" as maneuvers in the field of struggle over community health. While community health programs often embrace broad structural critiques and point to the social determinants of health as critical factors in health disparities, they frequently operate within constraints that force their attention instead to the level of individual behavior. In addition to offering a pragmatic approach to negotiation, asking for everything may be a productive way to think about collective organizing to solve problems of health inequality and access. What are the possibilities, from an identity-based approach to organizing (i.e., "by and for the community"), that are opened by asking for everything?

While community health programs may differ dramatically from grassroots social movements, they share some of the same challenges. Programs such as those discussed here struggle for legitimacy, to achieve community representation, to win regular and sustainable funding, and to serve target populations that are constructed or "known" through public health and ethnographic research. They run interventions seeking to prevent HIV, treat addiction, eliminate prejudice from health care, and bring the uninsured into the clinic. Through funding requirements such as those seen in Chapter 3, they are accountable to modes of economic rationality that transform nonprofit work using the language of "outcomes," "results," and "investments." Community health programs produce assemblages that bring together diverse forces: for example, harm reduction organizations find themselves working closely with police officers and becoming more tightly bound up with agencies of the state than they ever imagined possible, or desirable.

As these assemblages develop, discourses of community participation migrate from nonprofit helping agencies to help facilitate dramatic transformations in social benefit eligibility such as welfare reform. This process, which began in the 1970s, is ongoing, both in the United States and elsewhere (Clarke 2008). At the same time, the mobilizations of affected people and their advocates toward "universal values" such as health (Laclau 1995) produce powerful transformations in marginalized groups' self-understandings and new subject-positions from which political and health-related claims may be launched.

Community health interventions have wide-ranging and often unintended effects. The field of community health has become a crucial set of practices of government in which populations are constituted through their difference and by which they can be more effectively administered. In its focus on populations designated as urban, minority, or poor, community health engages in pragmatic activities as well as discursive practices that obscure the structural conditions constituting them as marginalized by use of the term *community*. Funded primarily by the state and nonprofit groups, HIV prevention and public health outreach programs administer these populations through concepts such as *empowerment* and *outreach*. Members of these groups are enlisted in practices of individual and collective self-management and self-government.[1]

---

1. The diffusion of the language of "community participation" and "empowerment" into diverse realms of governing has become even more widespread since the late 1990s. Beyond the federal welfare reform programs described here, empowerment has become

In a related process, advocates, including community health workers and experts, strive to develop a language and method for expanded access as they push for health care reform on both state and national levels to reach and enroll the so-called hardest-to-serve. Conceived as a way to form stronger links between health care providers and those in need of their services, community health outreach workers like the CHAs discussed in Part I are an example of community participation that emerged in response to the disenfranchisement of marginalized urban communities in the United States (Loyd 2010). Others, however, recognize the potential for discourses of community participation to serve as a terrain of government, where concerns about health care costs contend with a notion of citizenship that includes the right to health care.

Might community health programs do something differently to avoid or mitigate these governing effects? This question gets to the heart of the unique challenges facing applied anthropology, the effort to put anthropological ways of understanding to work solving pressing social problems. What can we learn from the successes and failures of these programs and the ways that they are implemented? In documenting diverse programs that aim to reduce inequality, I show how our very ideas of what constitutes "difference" or "the Other" are in fact defined by such programs. Rather than generating additional programmatic recommendations for policy makers and program designers, I instead reveal how these efforts are already unavoidably integrated with modes of neoliberal governance. As others have shown, even simply partaking in the language of empowerment invokes the interest of the state in having empowered citizens—now understood as those who are self-sufficient, middle-class consumers (e.g., Cruikshank 1999). While these relations of governing shape the conditions within which collective action takes place, the case studies discussed here illustrate the diverse ways in which community health programs affect both population health and individual and collective subjectivities.

The social relations of community, buttressed by structures of identification that link individuals with groups, offer important resources for action. In Gerald Creed's words, "*Community is an aspiration envisioned as an entity*" (Creed 2006b, 22, italics in original). What if we eschew the entity and continue to pursue the aspiration, with full knowledge of the constraints posed by economics, the state, and even the restrictive constructions of identity? What kinds of relations of community can we aspire to? Despite generations of critique of the concept by scholars from many disciplines, "community [remains] one of the most motivating discourses and practices circulating in contemporary society," eliciting "the strongest

---

standard operating procedure in international development programs (Sharma 2008; Leve 2007; Laurie, Andolina, and Radcliffe 2005), economic and community development in the United States and abroad (J. Stein 2000; Cruikshank 1999; Gupta and Sharma 2006), and public health (Lorway, Reza-Paul, and Pasha 2009; Israel et al. 2005).

of passions" (Joseph 2002, xxx). The case studies presented here explore several articulations of community as it contributes to the field of community health. In her important book, *Against the Romance of Community*, Miranda Joseph shows how meanings of community are supplementary to capital's demands for consumer behavior. She calls instead for "productive participation in collective action" that is "articulated as resistance or even [in] opposition to the flows of capital" (2002, 172). Such collective action might take many forms, providing opportunities for new forms of sociality and new alliances to emerge. In settings like Thornton's inner city, the liberatory possibilities of community relationships hold special potential as ways to mitigate the forces of marginalization. Joseph argues in favor of movements that are "potentially disruptive and displacing" of capital's relentless drive to produce communities as sites of affective bonding that foster appropriate consumption (2002, 172). In an earlier paper, Gerald Creed proposes a "notion of community in which conflict, both intra- and interethnic, is elemental and constitutive. This image of community does not demand consensus or homogeneity when imagined on a national scale" (2004, 56). Community health staffers and local activists articulate, as they try to mobilize, relations of community which already embody these elements of both conflict *and* identity. I follow both Loyd 2010 and Joseph 2002 in calling for community mobilization that is both reflexive and disruptive of its role as supplementary to capital, intervening in diverse political and institutional realms to realize actual social change.

As shown in the case studies presented here, community groups seeking to represent specific populations act on issues around community health as a practice of government, in part as a way to constitute themselves and to win more resources for their groups. Claims about need, health disparities, or the relevance of harm reduction for HIV prevention, for example, all have the effect of instantiating marginalized groups as political actors with voices that must be heeded. Recognition of these claims (Fraser 2001) contributes to the public visibility of a group and accelerates the process of individual identification with its collective aims, which drives a social movement and its representative organizations.

As seen in Part II, harm reduction activists witnessing the devastating AIDS epidemic among injection drug users (IDUs) seized the moment to call for and implement syringe exchange programs (SEPs) for IDUs as part of a broader harm reduction approach to drug use and addiction. As they achieved success after success, SEPs became entangled in new regimes of accountability imposed by more established funders.[2] Each of the groups discussed here—community-based public health workers, advocates for

---

2. The December 2009 overturning of the congressional ban on federal funding for syringe exchange should provide additional resources to SEPs, which can expect to find themselves accountable to ever new modes of surveillance and supervision as they receive federal funding.

culturally appropriate health care, and harm reduction groups—underwent similar processes of institutionalization as a result of the success of their advocacy efforts. Their interventions pulled each of these advocacy groups, previously constituted as an outsider social movement, into the assemblage of community health, propelling the governmental effects of their activism to new levels.

Difference may also offer a resource to those striving for greater recognition and access to care. Through the 1990s and 2000s, minority advocacy groups helped push the concept of health disparities into the headlines as a way to comment on and contest their marginalized status in U.S. society. As the concept of health disparities has gained political traction, efforts to attain recognition on the basis of difference must battle a countervailing democratic tendency against what is perceived as *special treatment* of one group over another. At the same time, this democratic belief in equality drives health disparities discourse and provides political grounding for the legitimacy of claimants seeking remedies for discrimination.

A similarly anxious ambivalence could be seen in popular debates around health care reform in the United States in 2009, where liberal anger at exclusion from the right to health care vied with populist and neoconservative resistance to the expansion of government in the Obama administration's proposed "public option," a publicly funded health insurance program (Espo 2009). Health care in the United States, and Americans' devotion to it, remains resolutely focused on both individual responsibility (in maintaining health and in ability to pay) and private profit. Despite enormously high rates of uninsurance (up to one in three U.S. residents in a given year [Bailey 2009]), and despite ongoing efforts at state and national reforms, employer-based health care continues to reign supreme. Americans seem to desire equality of access and outcomes while simultaneously favoring profits for health care delivery and the survival of the economically fittest. Even with the limited successes of those seeking to contest inequality by highlighting health disparities, a broader understanding of health care as a right has not perfused the popular media or town halls. In fact, when changes to the private employer-based system were proposed, Americans rallied in defense of private profit in the guise of "choice," "competition," and the desire for "privacy" between patients and their doctors.

In the face of such fervent commitment to an individualized, capitalist status quo, minority advocacy groups drawing attention to health disparities face an uphill battle in their call for cultural competence interventions for health care providers. Their allies include antiracist and immigrant advocacy groups who, in concert with medical education providers, are developing online and other educational programs for health care professionals. Cultural competence interventions aim to transform medical practices, the subjectivity of health care providers, and the meaning of difference as they present models of ethnicity and culture to health care providers as operative guides for practice.

New kinds of subjects emerge through these transformations: the active citizen, the ethically self-reflexive health care provider, the ethnically identified patient, the responsible drug user. In the process, communities demonstrate increased "capacity" by identifying problems and seeking resources to solve them, all apart from state bureaucracy. Individuals and communities both take part in and resist new modes of governing. In this way, the pragmatics and practices of neoliberal government are both ethical and teleological. Citizen-subjects collectively advocate for or against new programs and forms of entitlement based in part on their beliefs about what constitutes a just society, what the state's obligations are to its citizens, and who counts as a citizen. Implementing the programs that result from these struggles and transformations calls into being new subject-positions through discursive practices such as risk communication or empowerment-based education.

As epidemiological and ethnographic research transforms individuals' and groups' understanding of themselves as being "at risk" for HIV, harm reduction activists also work to bring forth new forms of identification among IDUs enrolled in SEPs. Harm reduction workers have both embraced these epidemiological risk categories and contested the "disease" paradigm of addiction and risk through concepts of "controlled use." By enrolling in SEPs, users are encouraged to take care of their communities at the same time that they are taking care of themselves. These moves are designed to foster drug users' identification with larger formations of community. Like the Community Health Advocate program described in Part I, community health programs seek to achieve transformations in subjectivity and foster the collective identification of problems facing economically and ethically marginalized groups. As activists, advocates, and researchers documenting these transformations, anthropologists face unique challenges in making our research legible in wider domains to support the liberatory aims of community health while critically examining the larger contexts and effects of these endeavors.

In contemporary U.S. society, struggles over community health are struggles over the nature and meaning of difference. *Difference* here can mean the condition of being underserved or in need; being outside the body politic; or being marked as poor, urban, or a racial or ethnic minority. Drawing their disciplinary expertise from biomedicine and public health, community health experts consider health on a population level. They develop a medicalized gaze aimed at the margins of society, generalizing across individuals to construct populations deemed most *at risk*. Their proposed interventions intersect with collective decisions made at the local level. Citizenship, community, access, and justice (e.g., are drug users criminals to be incarcerated or addicts in need of treatment?) are thus subject to popular contestation on the street, in the clinic, and at the ballot box. Both experts and citizen-subjects mobilize and generate concepts of difference as they diagnose problems, propose remedies, and work to make a world more receptive to justice and equality. These efforts contribute to a vision of empowerment that is able to criticize the conditions of its own possibility while engaging with others in pursuit of our mutual concerns.

References

Abel, David. 2005. "Westport Reverses Needle-Exchange Vote." *Boston Globe*, April 29. Available at http://www.boston.com/news/local/articles/2005/04/29/westport_reverses_needle_exchange_vote/.

Abramovitz, Mimi D. 1988. *Regulating the Lives of Women: Social Welfare Policy from Colonial Times to the Present*. Boston: South End Press.

Agar, Michael. 2002. "How the Drug Field Turned My Beard Grey." *International Journal of Drug Policy* 13 (4): 249–258.

Altman, Lawrence K. 2008. "Seeking Better Laws on HIV." *New York Times*, August 9, 11.

Anderson, Joan M., Sannie Tang, and Connie Blue. 2007. "Health Care Reform and the Paradox of Efficiency: 'Writing in' Culture." *International Journal of Health Services* 37 (2): 291–320.

Anderson, Laurie M., Susan Scrimshaw, Mindy Fullilove, Jonathan E. Fielding, Jacques Normand, and Task Force on Community Preventive Services. 2003. "Culturally Competent Healthcare Systems: A Systematic Review." *American Journal of Preventative Medicine* 24 (3S): 68–79.

Apter, David F., Herbert J. Gans, Ruth Horowitz, Gerald D. Jaynes, William Kornblum, Jr., James F. Short, Gerald D. Suttles, and Robert E. Washington. 2009. "The Chicago School and the Roots of Urban Ethnography: An Intergenerational Conversation with Gerald D. Jaynes, David E. Apter, Herbert J. Gans, William Kornblum, Ruth Horowitz, James F. Short, Jr., Gerald D. Suttles and Robert F. Washington." *Ethnography* 10 (4): 375–396.

Bailey, Kim. 2009. *Americans at Risk: One in Three Uninsured*. Washington, DC: Families USA.

Bane, Mary Jo, and D. David Ellwood. 1994. *Welfare Realities: From Rhetoric to Reform*. Cambridge, MA: Harvard University Press.

Barnett, Clive. 2005. "The Consolations of 'Neoliberalism.'" *Geoforum* 36:7–12.

Bastos, Francisco Inacio, and Steffanie Strathdee. 2000. "Evaluating Effectiveness of Syringe Exchange Programmes: Current Issues and Future Prospects." *Social Science and Medicine* 51 (12): 1771–1782.

Beach, M. C., E. G. Price, T. L. Gary, K. A. Robinson, A. Gozu, A. Palacio, C. Smarth, M. W. Jenckes, C. Feuerstein, E. B. Bass, N. R. Powe, and L. A. Cooper. 2005. "Cultural Competence: A Systematic Review of Health Care Provider Educational Interventions." *Med Care* 43 (4): 356–373.

Beam, Nancy, and Irene Tessaro. 1994. "The Lay Health Advisor Model in Theory and Practice: An Example of an Agency-Based Program." *Family and Community Health* 17 (3): 70–79.

Benjamin, Alan. 1999. "Contract and Covenant in Curacao." In *Beyond Regulations: Ethics in Human Subjects Research*, edited by N. King, G. Henderson, and J. Stein, 49–66. Chapel Hill: University of North Carolina Press.

Bennett, Tony. 2003. "Culture and Governmentality." In *Foucault, Cultural Studies, and Governmentality*, edited by J. Z. Bratich, J. Packer, and C. McCarthy, 47–65. Albany: SUNY Press.

Berger, Michele Tracy. 2004. *Workable Sisterhood: The Political Journey of Stigmatized Women with HIV/AIDS*. Princeton, NJ: Princeton University Press.

Biehl, João. 2004. "The Activist State: Global Pharmaceuticals, AIDS, and Citizenship in Brazil." *Social Text* 22 (3): 105–132.

———. 2005. "Technologies of Invisibility: Politics of Life and Social Inequality." In *Anthropologies of Modernity: Foucault, Governmentality, and Life Politics*, edited by J. X. Inda, 248–271. Malden, MA: Blackwell.

———. 2007. *Will to Live: AIDS Therapies and the Politics of Survival*. Princeton, NJ: Princeton University Press.

Bliss, Catherine. 2009. "Genome Sampling and the Biopolitics of Race." In *A Foucault for the 21st Century: Governmentality, Biopolitics and Discipline in the New Millennium*, edited by S. Binkley and J. Capetillo, 322–339. Boston, MA: Cambridge Scholars.

———. 2010. "Census, Race and Genomics." *Anthropology News* 51 (5): 9, 12.

Bluthenthal, Ricky. 1998. "Syringe Exchange as a Social Movement: A Case Study of Harm Reduction in Oakland, California." *Substance Use and Misuse* 33 (5): 1147–1171.

Bluthenthal, Ricky, Keith Heinzerling, Rachel Anderson, Neil Flynn, and Alex Kral. 2008. "Approval of Syringe Exchange Programs in California: Results from a Local Approach to HIV Prevention." *American Journal of Public Health* 98 (2): 278–283.

Bluthenthal, Ricky N., Greg Ridgeway, Terry Schell, Rachel Anderson, Neil M. Flynn, and Alex H. Kral. 2007. "Examination of the Association between Syringe Exchange Program (SEP) Dispensation Policy and SEP Client-Level Syringe Coverage among Injection Drug Users." *Addiction* 102 (4): 638–646.

Borovoy, Amy, and Janet Hine. 2008. "Managing the Unmanageable: Elderly Jewish Emigrés and the Biomedical Culture of Diabetes Care." *Medical Anthropology Quarterly* 22 (1): 1–26.

Bourdieu, Pierre. 1991. *Language and Symbolic Power*. Cambridge, MA: Harvard University Press.

Bourgois, Philippe. 1995. *In Search of Respect: Selling Crack in El Barrio*. Cambridge: Cambridge University Press.

———. 2000. "Disciplining Addictions: The Bio-politics of Methadone and Heroin in the United States." *Culture, Medicine and Psychiatry* 24:165–195.

————. 2002. "Anthropology and Epidemiology on Drugs: The Challenges of Cross-Methodological and Theoretical Dialogue." *International Journal of Drug Policy* 13:259–269.

————. 2009. *Righteous Dopefiend*. Berkeley: University of California Press.

Bourgois, Philippe, and Julie Bruneau. 2000. "Needle Exchange, HIV Infection, and the Politics of Science: Confronting Canada's Cocaine Injection Epidemic with Participant Observation." *Medical Anthropology* 18:325–350.

Braithwaite, Ronald, Cynthia Bianchi, and Sandra Taylor. 1994. "Ethnographic Approach to Community Organization and Empowerment." *Health Education Quarterly* 21 (3): 407–416.

Braithwaite, Ronald, Frederick Murphy, Ngina Lythcott, and Daniel Blumenthal. 1989. "Community Organization and Development for Health Promotion within an Urban Black Community: A Conceptual Model." *Health Education* 20 (5): 56–60.

Breines, Wini. 1989. *Community and Organization in the New Left, 1962–1968*. New Brunswick, NJ: Rutgers University Press.

Brettell, Caroline, ed. 1993. *When They Read What We Write: The Politics of Ethnography*. Westport, CT: Bergin and Garvey.

Briggs, Charles. 2003. "Why Nation-States and Journalists Can't Teach People to Be Healthy: Power and Pragmatic Miscalculation in Public Discourses on Health." *Medical Anthropology Quarterly* 17 (3): 287–321.

————. 2004. "Theorizing Modernity Conspiratorially: Science, Scale, and the Political Economy of Public Discourse in Explanations of a Cholera Epidemic." *American Ethnologist* 31 (2): 164–187.

Briggs, Charles, and Daniel Hallin. 2007. "Biocommunicability: The Neoliberal Subject and Its Contradictions in News Coverage of Health Issues." *Social Text* 25 (3): 43–66.

Broadhead, R., and Kathryn J. Fox. 1990. "Takin' It to the Streets: AIDS Outreach as Ethnography." *Journal of Contemporary Ethnography* 19 (3): 322–348.

Broadhead, R., Y. van Hulst, and D. Heckathorn. 1999. "Termination of an Established Needle-Exchange: A Study of Claims and their Impact." *Social Problems* 46 (1): 48–66.

Brodkin, Evelyn. 1997. "Inside the Welfare Contract: Discretion and Accountability in State Welfare Administration." *Social Service Review* 71 (1): 1–33.

Brownlie, Julie, and Alexandra Howson. 2006. "Between the Demands of Truth and Government: Health Practitioners, Trust and Immunisation Work." *Social Science and Medicine* 62 (2): 433–443.

Buchanan, David, Susan Shaw, Amy Ford, and Merrill Singer. 2004. "Empirical Science Meets Moral Panic: An Analysis of the Politics of Needle Exchange." *Journal of Health Politics, Policy and Law* 24 (3–4): 427–444.

Buchanan, David, Susan Shaw, Wei Teng, Poppy Hiser, and Merrill Singer. 2002. "Neighborhood Differences in Patterns of Syringe Access, Use and Discard: Implications for HIV Outreach and Prevention Education." *Journal of Urban Health* 80 (3): 438–454.

Bunton, Robin. 2005. *Genetic Governance: Health, Risk and Ethics in a Biotech Era*. London: Routledge.

Burchell, Graham. 1996. "Liberal Government and Techniques of the Self." In *Foucault and Political Reason*, edited by A. Barry, T. Osborne, and N. Rose, 19–36. Chicago: University of Chicago Press.

Butler, Judith. 1990. *Gender Trouble: Feminism and the Subversion of Identity*. New York: Routledge.

Campbell, Nancy. 1995. "Cold War Compulsions: U.S. Drug Science, Policy, and Culture." Ph.D. diss., History of Consciousness Program, University of California, Santa Cruz.

———. 2000. *Using Women: Gender, Drug Policy and Social Justice.* New York: Routledge.

———. 2007. *Discovering Addiction: The Science and Politics of Substance Abuse Research.* Ann Arbor: University of Michigan Press.

Campbell, Nancy, and Susan Shaw. 2008. "Incitements to Discourse: Illicit Drugs, Harm Reduction and the Production of Ethnographic Subjects." *Cultural Anthropology* 23 (4): 688–717.

Cant, Sarah, and Ursula Sharma. 1996. "Demarcation and Transformation within Homeopathic Knowledge: A Strategy of Professionalization." *Social Science and Medicine* 42 (4): 579–588.

Carlen, Pat. 2008. "Imaginary Penalities and Risk-Crazed Governance." In *Imaginary Penalities*, edited by P. Carlen, 1–25. Portland, OR: Willan.

Carr, Summerson. 2009. "Anticipating and Inhabiting Institutional Identities." *American Ethnologist* 36 (2): 317–336.

Castel, Robert. 1991. "From Dangerousness to Risk." In *The Foucault Effect: Studies in Governmentality*, edited by G. Burchell, C. Gordon, and P. Miller, 281–298. Chicago: University of Chicago Press.

Caughey, John. 1986. "On the Anthropology of America." In *Symbolizing America*, edited by H. Varenne, 229–250. Lincoln: University of Nebraska Press.

Chapman, Rachel R., and Jean R. Berggren. 2005. "Radical Contextualization: Contributions to an Anthropology of Racial/Ethnic Health Disparities." *Health* 9 (2): 145–167.

Clarke, John. 2007. "Unsettled Connections: Citizen, Consumers and the Reform of Public Services." *Journal of Consumer Culture* 7 (2): 159–178.

———. 2008. "Reconstructing Nation, State and Welfare: The Transformation of Welfare States." In *Welfare State Transformations: Comparative Perspectives*, edited by M. Seelieb-Kaiser, 197–209. Basingstoke, UK: Palgrave Macmillan.

Clarke, Kamari Maxine, and Deborah Thomas, eds. 2006. *Globalization and Race: Transformation in the Cultural Production of Blackness.* Durham, NC: Duke University Press.

Clatts, Michael. 1995. "Disembodied Acts: On the Perverse Use of Sexual Categories in the Study of High-Risk Behavior." In *Culture and Sexual Risk: Anthropological Perspectives*, edited by H. ten Brummelhuis and G. Herdt, 241–256. New York: Gordon and Breach.

Collie, Tim. 2001. "Needle Exchanges Help Save Lives in Puerto Rico." [South Florida] *Sun-Sentinel*, July 8, 1A.

Collier, Stephen J., and Andrew Lakoff. 2005. "On Regimes of Living." In *Global Assemblages: Technology, Politics, and Ethics as Anthropological Problems*, edited by A. Ong and S. J. Collier, 22–39. Malden, MA: Blackwell.

Collier, Stephen J., and Aihwa Ong. 2005. "Global Assemblages, Anthropological Problems." In *Global Assemblages: Technology, Politics, and Ethics as Anthropological Problems*, edited by A. Ong and S. J. Collier, 3–21. Malden, MA: Blackwell.

Comaroff, John L., and Jean Comaroff. 2009. *Ethnicity, Inc.* Chicago: University of Chicago Press.

Creed, Gerald. 2004. "Constituted through Conflict: Images of Community (and Nation) in Bulgarian Rural Ritual." *American Anthropologist* 106 (1): 56–70.

————. 2006a. "Community as Modern Pastoral." In *The Seductions of Community: Emancipations, Oppressions, Quandaries*, edited by G. Creed, 23–48. Santa Fe, NM: School of American Research.

————, ed. 2006b. *The Seductions of Community: Emancipations, Oppressions, Quandaries*. Santa Fe, NM: School of American Research.

Crehan, Kate. 2006. "Hunting the Unicorn: Art and Community in East London." In *The Seductions of Community: Emancipations, Oppressions, Quandaries*, edited by G. Creed, 49–76. Santa Fe, NM: School of American Research.

Crenshaw, Kimberlé, Neil Gotanda, Gary Peller, and Kendall Thomas, eds. 1995. *Critical Race Theory: The Key Writings That Formed the Movement*. New York: New Press/Norton.

Cruikshank, Barbara. 1999. *The Will to Empower: Democratic Citizens and Other Subjects*. Ithaca, NY: Cornell University Press.

Davis, Dana Ain. 2006. "Knowledge in the Service of a Vision: Politically Engaged Anthropology." In *Engaged Observer: Anthropology, Advocacy and Activism*, edited by V. Sanford and A. Angel-Ajani, 228–238. New Brunswick, NJ: Rutgers University.

Davis, Mark, and Tim Rhodes. 2004. "Managing Seen and Unseen Blood Associated with Drug Injecting: Implications for Theorising Harm Reduction for Viral Risk." *International Journal of Drug Policy* 15:377–384.

Dean, Mitchell. 1997. "Governing the Unemployed Self in an Active Society." *Economy and Society* 24 (4): 559–583.

————. 1999. *Governmentality: Power and Rule in Modern Society*. London: Sage.

de la Cadena, Marisol. 2000. *Indigenous Mestizos: The Politics of Race and Culture in Cuzco 1919–1991*. Durham, NC: Duke University Press.

Deleuze, Gilles, and Felix Guattari. 1987. *A Thousand Plateaus: Capitalism and Schizophrenia*. Translated by B. Massumi. Minneapolis: University of Minnesota Press.

D'Emilio, John. 2003. "The Gay Liberation Movement." In *The Social Movement Reader: Cases and Concepts*, edited by J. Goodwin and J. Jasper, 32–37. Malden, MA: Blackwell.

Denny, Keith. 1999. "Evidence-Based Medicine and Medical Authority." *Journal of Medical Humanities* 20 (4): 247–263.

Deren, Sherry, Charles Cleland, Crystal Fuller, Sung-Yeon Kang, Don Des Jarlais, and David Vlahov. 2006. "The Impact of Syringe Deregulation on Sources of Syringes for Injection Drug Users: Preliminary Findings." *AIDS and Behavior* 10 (6): 717–721.

Des Jarlais, Donald, Kamyar Arasteh, Holly Hagan, Courtney McKnight, David Perlman, and Samuel Friedman. 2009. "Persistence and Change in Disparities in HIV Infection among Injection Drug Users in New York City after Large-Scale Syringe Exchange Programs." *American Journal of Public Health* 99 (Suppl. 2): S445–451.

diLeonardo, Micaela. 2006. "There's No Place Like Home: Domestic Domains and Urban Imaginaries in New Haven, Connecticut." *Identities: Global Studies in Culture and Power* 13 (1): 33–52.

Donovan, Mark C. 1996. "The Politics of Deservedness: The Ryan White Act and the Social Constructions of People with AIDS." In *AIDS: The Politics and Policy of Disease*, edited by S. Z. Theodoulou, 68–87. Upper Saddle River, NJ: Prentice Hall.

Dressler, William, Kathryn Oths, and Clarence Gravlee. 2005. "Race and Ethnicity in Public Health Research: Models to Explain Health Disparities." *Annual Review of Anthropology* 34:231–252.

Duff, Cameron. 2004. "Drug Use as a 'Practice of the Self': Is There Any Place for an 'Ethics of Moderation' in Contemporary Drug Policy?" *International Journal of Drug Policy* 15:385–393.

Duggan, Lisa. 2004. *The Twilight of Equality: Neoliberalism, Cultural Politics, and the Attack on Democracy.* Boston, MA: Beacon Press.

Earp, Joanne, Claire Viadro, Amy Vincus, Mary Altpeter, Valerie Flax, Linda Mayne, and Eugenia Eng. 1997. "Lay Health Advisors: A Strategy for Getting the Word Out about Breast Cancer." *Health Education and Behavior* 24 (4): 432–451.

Egelko, Bob. 2009. "U.S. Repeals Funding Ban for Needle Exchanges." *San Francisco Chronicle*, December 17, A126.

Eiserman, Julie, Claudia Santelices, Anna Marie Nicolaysen, Thomas Stopka, and Merrill Singer. 2003. "What Do They Mean, When They Say Clean? When They Say New? Examining the Complexity of Injection Drug Users' Descriptions of Syringes Purchased from the Street." Paper presented at Turning Research into Prevention: The National HIV Prevention Conference, Centers for Disease Control and Prevention, Atlanta, August 13.

Eng, Eugenia, Edith Parker, and Christina Harlan. 1997. "Lay Health Advisor Intervention Strategies: A Continuum from Natural Helping to Paraprofessional Helping." *Health Education and Behavior* 24 (4): 413–417.

Eng, Eugenia, and Rebecca Young. 1992. "Lay Health Advisors as Community Change Agents." *Family and Community Health* 15 (1): 24–40.

Epstein, Steven. 1996. *Impure Science.* Berkeley: University of California Press.

———. 2007. *Inclusion: The Politics of Difference in Medical Research.* Chicago: University of Chicago Press.

Erickson, Patricia, Diane Riley, Yuet Cheung, and Pat O'Hare, eds. 1997. *Harm Reduction: A New Direction for Drug Policies and Programs.* Toronto: University of Toronto Press.

Escobar, Arturo, Dianne Rocheleau, and Smitu Kothari. 2002. "Environmental Social Movements and the Politics of Place." *Development* 45 (1): 28–37.

Espo, David. 2009. "Few Favor Health Care Concession; Possible Dropping of 'Public Option' Angers Liberals, Gets Little Republican Support." *Chicago Sun-Times*, August 18, 14.

Ess, Charles, and the Association of Internet Researchers. 2002. "Ethical Decision-Making and Internet Research: Recommendations from the AOIR Ethics Working Committee." Available at http://aoir.org/reports/ethics.pdf.

Ettore, Elizabeth. 2004. "Revisioning Women and Drug Use: Gender Sensitivity, Embodiment and Reducing Harm." *International Journal of Drug Policy* 15: 327–335.

Fairchild, Amy L., Ronald Bayer, and James Colgrove. 2007. *Searching Eyes: Privacy, the State, and Disease Surveillance in America.* Berkeley: University of California Press.

Farmer, Paul. 1992. *AIDS and Accusation: Haiti and the Geography of Blame.* Berkeley: University of California Press.

Fassin, Didier. 2007. *When Bodies Remember: Experiences and Politics of AIDS in South Africa.* Berkeley: University of California Press.

Fausto-Sterling, Anne. 2004. "Refashioning Race: DNA and the Politics of Health Care." *Differences: A Journal of Feminist Cultural Studies* 15 (3): 1–37.

Feinstein, Alvan R., and Ralph I. Horwitz. 1997. "Problems in the 'Evidence' of 'Evidence-Based Medicine.'" *American Journal of Medicine* 103 (6): 529–535.

Feldman, Allen. 2001. "Philoctetes Revisited: White Public Space and the Political Geography of Public Safety." *Social Text* 19 (3): 57–89.

Feldman, Harvey W., and Patrick Biernacki. 1988. "The Ethnography of Needle Sharing among Intravenous Drug Users and Implications for Public Policies and Intervention Strategies." In *Needle-Sharing among Intravenous Drug Abusers: National and International Perspectives*, edited by R. J. Battjes and R. W. Pickens, 28–39. Washington, DC: NIDA Research Monograph Series.

Ferguson, James. 1994. *The Anti-Politics Machine: Development, Depoliticization, and Bureaucratic Power in Lesotho*. Minneapolis: University of Minnesota Press.

Ferguson, James, and Akhil Gupta. 2002. "Spatializing States: Toward an Ethnography of a Neoliberal Governmentality." *American Ethnologist* 4 (28): 981–1002.

Finn, Janet, and Lyne Underwood. 2000. "The State, the Clock, and the Struggle: An Inquiry into the Discipline for Welfare Reform in Montana." *Social Text* 18 (1): 109–134.

Fischer, Benedikt, and Blake Poland. 1998. "Exclusion, 'Risk,' and Social Control: Reflections on Community Policing and Public Health." *Geoforum* 29 (2): 187–197.

Fischer, Benedikt, Sarah Turnbull, Blake Poland, and Emma Haydon. 2004. "Drug Use, Risk, and Urban Order: Examining Supervised Injection Sites (SIS) as 'Governmentality.'" *International Journal of Drug Policy* 15 (5–6): 357–365.

Forman, Shepard, ed. 1995. *Diagnosing America: Anthropology and Public Engagement*. Ann Arbor: University of Michigan Press.

Foucault, Michel. 1975. *The Birth of the Clinic: An Archaeology of Medical Perception*. New York: Random House.

———. 1978. *The History of Sexuality: Introduction*. Vol. 1. New York: Vintage Books.

———. 1991. "Governmentality." In *The Foucault Effect: Studies in Governmentality*, edited by G. Burchell, C. Gordon, and P. Miller, 87–104. Chicago: University of Chicago Press.

Frankenberg, Ruth. 1993. *The Social Construction of Whiteness: White Women, Race Matters*. Minneapolis: University of Minnesota Press.

Fraser, Nancy. 1989. *Unruly Practices: Power, Discourse and Gender in Contemporary Social Theory*. Minneapolis: University of Minnesota Press.

———. 2001. "Recognition without Ethics?" *Theory, Culture and Society* 18 (2–3): 21–42.

Fraser, Nancy, and Linda Gordon. 1994. "The Genealogy of Dependency: Tracing a Keyword of the U.S. Welfare State." *Signs* 19:309–336.

Freire, Paulo. 1974. *Pedagogy of the Oppressed*. New York: Seabury Press.

Fullilove, M., A. Lown, and R. E. Fullilove. 1992. "Crack 'Hos and Skeezers: Traumatic Experiences of Women Crack Users." *Journal of Sex Research* 29 (2): 275–287.

Fullilove, Mindy Thompson. 2001. "Root Shock: The Consequences of African-American Dispossession." *Journal of Urban Health* 78 (1): 72–80.

Fullwiley, Duana. 2007. "Race and Genetics: Attempts to Define the Relationship." *BioSocieties* 2 (2): 221–237.

Garcia, Angela. 2010. *The Pastoral Clinic: Addiction and Dispossession along the Rio Grande*. Berkeley: University of California Press.

Gastaldo, Denise. 1997. "Health Education and the Concept of Biopower." In *Foucault, Health and Medicine*, edited by A. Petersen and R. Bunton, 113–133. London: Routledge.

Geary, Adam M. 2007. "Culture as an Object of Ethical Governance in AIDS Prevention." *Cultural Studies* 21 (4–5): 672–694.

Giddens, Anthony. 1994. "Living in a Post-traditional Society." In *Reflexive Modernization: Politics, Tradition and Aesthetics in the Modern Social Order*, edited by U. Beck, A. Giddens, and S. Lash, 56–109. Cambridge, UK: Polity Press.

Gilbert, Neil. 2002. *Transformation of the Welfare State: The Silent Surrender of Public Responsibility*. Oxford, UK: Oxford University Press.

Gilliom, John. 1997. "Everyday Surveillance, Everyday Resistance: Computer Monitoring in the Lives of the Appalachian Poor." *Studies in Law, Politics and Society* 16:275–297.

Gilroy, Paul. 1993. *The Black Atlantic: Modernity and Double Consciousness*. Cambridge, MA: Harvard University Press.

Glick Schiller, Nina, Stephen Crystal, and Denver Lewellen. 1994. "Risky Business: The Cultural Construction of AIDS Risk Groups." *Social Science and Medicine* 38 (10): 1337–1346.

Good, Byron, and Mary-Jo Good. 1993. "Learning Medicine: The Constructing of Medical Knowledge at Harvard Medical School." In *Knowledge, Power and Practice*, edited by S. Lindenbaum and M. Lock, 81–107. Berkeley: University of California Press.

Good, Mary-Jo DelVecchio, Sarah S. Willen, Seth Donal Hannah, Ken Vickery, and Lawrence T. Park. 2011. *Shattering Culture: American Medicine Responds to Cultural Diversity*. New York: Russell Sage Foundation.

Goode, Judith. 2001. "Let's Get Our Act Together: How Racial Discourses Disrupt Neighborhood Activism." In *The New Poverty Studies: The Ethnography of Power, Politics and Impoverished People in the United States*, edited by Judith Goode and Jeff Maskovsky, 364–398. New York: New York University Press.

Goode, Judith, and Jeff Maskovsky. 2001. "Introduction." In *The New Poverty Studies: The Ethnography of Power, Politics and Impoverished People in the United States*, edited by Judith Goode and Jeff Maskovsky, 1–34. New York: New York University Press.

Goodman, R. M., M. A. Speers, K. McLeroy, S. Fawcett, M. Kegler, E. Parker, S. R. Smith, T. D. Sterling, and N. Wallerstein. 1998. "Identifying and Defining the Dimensions of Community Capacity to Provide a Basis for Measurement." *Health Education and Behavior* 25 (3): 258–278.

Gordon, Linda, ed. 1990. *Women, the State, and Welfare*. Madison: University of Wisconsin Press.

Gravlee, Clarence, and Elizabeth Sweet. 2008. "Race, Ethnicity, and Racism in Medical Anthropology, 1977–2002." *Medical Anthropology Quarterly* 22 (1): 27–51.

Gupta, Akhil, and James Ferguson. 1997. "Beyond 'Culture': Space, Identity and the Politics of Difference." In *Culture, Power, Place: Explorations in Critical Identity*, edited by A. Gupta and J. Ferguson, 33–51. Durham, NC: Duke University Press.

Gupta, Akhil, and Aradhana Sharma. 2006. "Globalization and Postcolonial States." *Current Anthropology* 47 (2): 277–307.

Hacking, Ian. 1986. "Making Up People." In *Reconstructing Individualism: Autonomy, Individuality and the Self in Western Thought*, edited by Thomas Heller, Morton Sosna, and David Wellbery, 222–236. Stanford, CA: Stanford University Press.

Hagan, Holly, Donald Des Jarlais, and David Purchase. 1993. "An Interview Study of Participants in the Tacoma, Washington, Syringe Exchange." *Addiction* 88: 1691–1698.

Hannah, Seth. 2008. "Clinical Care in Environments of Hyperdiversity: Race, Culture, and Ethnicity in the Post-Pentad World." Paper presented at the conference Celebrating a Quarter Century of the Harvard NIMH Medical Anthropology Training Program, Harvard University, Cambridge, MA, May 16.

Harrison, Faye. 1991. "Ethnography as Politics." In *Decolonizing Anthropology: Moving Further toward an Anthropology for Liberation*, edited by Faye Harrison, 88–109. Washington, DC: American Anthropological Association.

Harvard School of Public Health. 2009. Diversitydata.org.

Harvey, Carol, and M. June Allard. 2004. *Understanding and Managing Diversity*. Englewood Cliffs, NJ: Prentice Hall.

Harvey, David. 2005. *A Brief History of Neoliberalism*. Oxford, UK: Oxford University Press.

Hasnain-Wynia, Romana. 2010. "Racial and Ethnic Disparities within and between Hospitals for Inpatient Quality of Care: An Examination of Patient-Level Hospital Quality Alliance Measures." *Journal of Health Care for the Poor and Underserved* 21 (2): 629–648.

Hay, M. Cameron, Thomas S. Weisner, Naihua Duan, Saskia Subramanian, Edward Nedenski, and Richard Kravitz. 2008. "Harnessing Experience: Exploring the Gap between Evidence Based Medicine and Clinical Practice." *Journal of Evaluation of Clinical Experience* 14 (5): 707–713.

Heath, Deborah, Rayna Rapp, and Karen-Sue Taussig. 2004. "Genetic Citizenship." In *A Companion to the Anthropology of Politics*, edited by David Nugent and Joan Vincent, 153–167. Malden, MA: Blackwell.

Heath, Melanie. 2009. "State of Our Unions: Marriage Promotion and the Contested Power of Heterosexuality." *Gender and Society* 1 (23): 27–48.

Heimer, Robert, Ricky Bluthenthal, Merrill Singer, and Kaveh Khoshnood. 1996. "Structural Impediments to Operational Syringe Exchange Programs." *AIDS and Public Policy Journal* 11:169–184.

Heimer, Robert, Kaveh Khoshnood, Dan Bigg, J. Guydish, and B. Junge. 1998. "Syringe Use and Re-Use: Effects of Syringe Exchange Programs in Four Cities." *Journal of Acquired Immune Deficiency Syndromes and Human Retrovirology* 18 (Suppl. 1): S37–S44.

Heller, D. I., D. Paone, A. Siegler, and A. Karpati. 2009. "The Syringe Gap: An Assessment of Sterile Syringe Need and Acquisition among Syringe Exchange Program Participants in New York City." *Harm Reduction Journal* 6:1.

Hemment, Julie. 2007. *Empowering Women in Russia: Activism, Aid, and NGOs*. Bloomington: Indiana University Press.

Henman, A. R., D. Paone, D. C. Des Jarlais, L. M. Kochems, and S. R. Friedman. 1998. "Injection Drug Users as Social Actors: A Stigmatized Community's Participation in the Syringe Exchange Programmes of New York City." *AIDS Care* 10 (4): 397–408.

Herdt, Gil, and Shirley Lindenbaum, eds. 1992. *The Time of AIDS: Social Analysis, Theory, and Method*. Newbury Park, CA: Sage.

Hill, M. Anne, and Thomas J. Main. 1998. *Is Welfare Working? The Massachusetts Reforms Three Years Later*. Boston: Pioneer Institute for Public Policy Research.

Hogle, Linda F. 2002a. "Claims and Disclaimers: Whose Expertise Counts?" *Medical Anthropology Quarterly* 21 (3–4): 275–306.

———. 2002b. "Introduction: Jurisdictions of Authority and Expertise in Science and Medicine." *Medical Anthropology* 21 (3–4): 231–246.

Horton, Sarah, and Judith Barker. 2009. "'Stains' on Their Self-Discipline: Public Health, Hygiene, and the Disciplining of Undocumented Immigrant Parents in the Nation's Internal Borderlands." *American Ethnologist* 36 (4): 784–798.

Hyatt, Sue. 2001. "From Citizen to Volunteer: Neoliberal Governance and the Erasure of Poverty." In *The New Poverty Studies: The Ethnography of Power, Politics and Impoverished People in the United States*, edited by J. Goode and J. Maskovsky, 201–235. New York: New York University Press.

Igo, Sarah. 2007. *The Averaged American: Surveys, Citizens, and the Making of a Mass Public*. Cambridge, MA: Harvard University Press.

Ilcan, Suzan, and Tanya Basok. 2004. "Community Government: Voluntary Agencies, Social Justice, and the Responsibilization of Citizens." *Citizenship Studies* 8 (2): 129–144.

Inciardi, James A., and L. D. Harrison. 2000. *Harm Reduction: National and International Perspectives*. Newbury Park, CA: Sage.

Inda, Jonathan Xavier, ed. 2005. *Anthropologies of Modernity: Foucault, Governmentality, and Life Politics*. Malden, MA: Blackwell.

Institute of Medicine, Brian Smedley, Adrienne Y. Stith, and Alan R. Nelson. 2003. *Unequal Treatment: Confronting Racial and Ethnic Disparities in Health Care*. Washington, DC: National Academies Press.

Israel, B. A., E. A. Parker, Z. Rowe, A. Salvatore, M. Minkler, J. Lopez, A. Butz, A. Mosley, L. Coates, G. Lambert, P. A. Potito, B. Brenner, M. Rivera, H. Romero, B. Thompson, G. Coronado, and S. Halstead. 2005. "Community-Based Participatory Research: Lessons Learned from the Centers for Children's Environmental Health and Disease Prevention Research." *Environmental Health Perspectives* 113 (10): 1463–1471.

Israel, B. A., A. J. Schulz, E. A. Parker, and A. B. Becker. 1998. "Review of Community-Based Research: Assessing Partnership Approaches to Improve Public Health." *Annual Review of Public Health* 19:173–202.

Jencks, Stephen F., and Gail R. Wilensky. 1992. "The Health-Care Quality Improvement Initiative: A New Approach to Quality Assurance in Medicare." *Journal of the American Medical Association* 268 (7): 900–903.

Jenks, Angela. 2009. "'Cultural Competence' and the Medical Management of Difference." Ph.D. diss., Department of Anthropology, University of California, Berkeley.

———. 2011. "From 'Lists of Traits' to 'Open-Mindedness': Emerging Issues in Cultural Competence Education." *Culture, Medicine and Psychiatry* 35 (2): 209–235.

Jewett, Sarah. 2006. "'If You Don't Identify with Your Ancestry, You're Like a Race without a Land': Constructing Race at a Small Urban Middle School." *Anthropology and Education Quarterly* 37 (2): 144–161.

Jones, Matthew. 2004. "Anxiety and Containment in the Risk Society: Theorising Young People and Drug Prevention Policy." *International Journal of Drug Policy* 15:367–376.

Joseph, Miranda. 2002. *Against the Romance of Community*. Minneapolis: University of Minnesota Press.

Kahn, Jonathan. 2006. "Genes, Race, and Population: Avoiding a Collision of Categories." *American Journal of Public Health* 96 (11): 1965–1970.

Kane, Stephanie, and Theresa Mason. 1992. "'IV Drug Users' and 'Sex Partners': The Limits of Epidemiological Categories and the Ethnography of Risk." In *The Time of AIDS: Social Analysis, Theory, and Method*, edited by G. Herdt and S. Lindenbaum, 199–222. Newbury Park, CA: Sage.

Kark, Sydney, and Emily Kark. 1999. *Promoting Community Health: From Pholela to Jerusalem*. Johannesburg, South Africa: Witwatersrand University Press.

Kehoe, K. A., G. D. Melkus, and K. Newlin. 2003. "Culture within the Context of Care: An Integrative Review." *Ethnicity and Disease* 13 (3): 344–353.

Klawiter, Maren. 2008. *The Biopolitics of Breast Cancer: Changing Cultures of Disease and Activism*. Minneapolis: University of Minnesota Press.

Kleinman, Arthur. 1980. *Patients and Healers in the Context of Culture: An Exploration of the Borderland between Anthropology, Medicine, and Psychiatry*. Berkeley: University of California Press.

———. 1988. *The Illness Narratives: Suffering, Healing, and the Human Condition*. New York: Basic Books.

Kleinman, Arthur, and Peter Benson. 2006. "Anthropology in the Clinic: The Problem of Cultural Competency and How to Fix It." *PLoS Medicine (Public Library of Science)* 3 (10): 1673–1676.

Koch, Lene, and Mette Nordahl Svendsen. 2005. "Providing Solutions, Defining Problems: The Imperative of Disease in Prevention in Genetic Counselling." *Social Science and Medicine* 60 (4): 823–832.

Korteweg, Anna C. 2003. "Welfare Reform and the Subject of the Working Mother: 'Get a Job, a Better Job, Then a Career.'" *Theory and Society* 32 (4): 445–480.

Kottak, Conrad, and Kathryn Kozaitis. 2007. *On Being Different: Diversity and Multiculturalism in the North American Mainstream.* New York: McGraw-Hill.

Kramer, Frederica. 1998. "The Hard-to-Place: Understanding the Population and Strategies to Serve Them." *Welfare Information Network Issue Notes* 2 (5): 5–9.

Kretzmann, J. P., and J. L. McKnight. 1993. *Building Communities from the Inside Out: A Path toward Finding and Mobilizing a Community's Assets.* Chicago: ACTA.

Krieger, Nancy, Jarvis T. Chen, Pamela D. Waterman, David H. Rehkopf, and S. V. Subramanian. 2005. "Painting a Truer Picture of U.S. Socioeconomic and Racial/Ethnic Health Inequalities: The Public Health Disparities Geocoding Project." *American Journal of Public Health* 95 (2): 312–324.

Laclau, Ernesto. 1995. "Universalism, Particularism, and the Question of Identity." In *The Identity in Question*, edited by J. Rajchman, 93–110. New York: Routledge.

Laine, C., and F. Davidoff. 1996. "Patient-Centered Medicine: A Professional Evolution." *Journal of the American Medical Association* 275 (2): 152–156.

Lambert, Helen. 2006. "Accounting for EBM: Notions of Evidence in Medicine." *Social Science and Medicine* 62 (11): 2633–2645.

Larner, Wendy. 2005. "Neoliberalism in (Regional) Theory and Practice: The Stronger Communities Action Fund in New Zealand." *Geographical Research* 43 (1): 9–18.

Lash, Scott, Bronislaw Szerszynski, and Brian Wynne, eds. 1996. *Risk, Environment and Modernity.* London: Sage.

Lassiter, Luke Eric. 2005. "Collaborative Ethnography and Public Anthropology." *Current Anthropology* 46 (1): 83–106.

Latour, Bruno. 1988. *Science in Action.* Cambridge, MA: Harvard University Press.

Laurie, Nina, Robert Andolina, and Sarah Radcliffe. 2005. "Ethnodevelopment: Social Movements, Creating Experts and Professionalising Indigenous Knowledge in Ecuador." *Antipode* 37 (3): 470–496.

Lee, Simon Craddock. 2005. "The Risks of Race in Addressing Health Disparities." *Hastings Center Report* 35 (4): 49.

Lefkowitz, Bonnie. 2007. *Community Health Centers: A Movement and the People Who Made It Happen.* New Brunswick, NJ: Rutgers University Press.

Leslie, Deborah, and David Butz. 1998. "'GM Suicide': Flexibility, Space, and the Injured Body." *Economic Geography* 74 (4): 360–378.

Leve, Lauren. 2007. "'Failed Development' and Rural Revolution in Nepal: Rethinking Subaltern Consciousness and Women's Empowerment." *Anthropological Quarterly* 80 (1): 127–172.

Li, Tania Murray. 2005. "Beyond 'the State' and Failed Schemes." *American Anthropologist* 107 (3): 383–394.

———. 2007. *The Will to Improve: Governmentality, Development, and the Practice of Politics.* Durham, NC: Duke University Press.

Limoncelli, Stephanie. 2002. "Some of Us Are Excellent at Babies: Paid Work, Mothering, and the Construction of Need in a Welfare-to-Work Program." In *Work, Welfare and Politics: Confronting Poverty in the Wake of Welfare Reform,* edited by Frances Fox Piven, Joan Acker Margaret Hallock, and Sandra Morgen, 81–94. Eugene: University of Oregon Press.

Lindenbaum, Shirley. 1992. "Knowledge and Action in the Shadow of AIDS." In *The Time of AIDS: Social Analysis, Theory, and Method*, edited by G. Herdt and S. Lindenbaum, 319–334. Newbury Park, CA: Sage.

Little, Peter C. 2009. "Negotiating Community Engagement and Science in the Federal Environmental Public Health Sector." *Medical Anthropology Quarterly* 23 (2): 94–118.

Lorvick, Jennifer, Ricky N. Bluthenthal, Andrea Scott, Mary Lou Gilbert, Kara S. Riehman, Rachel L. Anderson, Neil M. Flynn, and Alex H. Kral. 2006. "Secondary Syringe Exchange among Users of 23 California Syringe Exchange Programs." *Substance Use and Misuse* 41 (6–7): 865–882.

Lorway, Robert, Sushena Reza-Paul, and Akram Pasha. 2009. "On Becoming a Male Sex Worker in Mysore: Sexual Subjectivity, 'Empowerment,' and Community-Based HIV Prevention Research." *Medical Anthropology Quarterly* 23 (2): 142–160.

Lovell, Anne. 2006. "Addiction Markets: The Case of High-Dose Buprenorphine in France." In *Global Pharmaceuticals: Ethics, Markets, Practices*, edited by A. Petryna, A. Lakoff, and A. Kleinman, 136–170. Durham, NC: Duke University Press.

Lovell, Anne, and Sandra Cohn. 1998. "The Elaboration of 'Choice' in a Program for Homeless Persons Labeled Psychiatrically Disabled." *Human Organization* 57 (1): 8–20.

Loyd, Jenne. 2010. "Where Is Community Health? Racism, the Clinic, and the Biopolitical State." In *Rebirth of the Clinic: Places and Agents in Contemporary Health Care*, edited by C. Patton, 39–67. Minneapolis: University of Minnesota Press.

Lubove, Roy. 1965. *The Professional Altruist: The Emergence of Social Work as a Career 1880–1930*. Cambridge, MA: Harvard University Press.

Lupton, Deborah. 1999. *Risk*. London: Routledge.

Lyon-Callo, Vincent. 2004. *Inequality, Poverty, and Neoliberal Governance: Activist Ethnography in the Homeless Sheltering Industry*. Peterborough, Canada: Broadview Press.

Lyon-Callo, Vincent, and Susan Hyatt. 2003. "The Neoliberal State and the Depoliticization of Poverty: Activist Anthropology and 'Ethnography from Below.'" *Urban Anthropology* 32 (2): 175–204.

Management Sciences for Health. n.d. "Common Beliefs and Cultural Practices: Pacific Islanders." *The Provider's Guide to Quality and Culture*. Available at http://erc.msh.org/mainpage.cfm?file=5.3.0f.htm&module=provider&language=English.

Manson, Spero M. 2003. "Extending the Boundaries, Bridging the Gaps: Crafting Mental Health: Culture, Race, and Ethnicity, a Supplement to the Surgeon General's Report on Mental Health." *Culture, Medicine and Psychiatry* 27 (4): 395–408.

Marinetto, Michael. 2003. "Who Wants to Be an Active Citizen? The Politics and Practice of Community Involvement." *Sociology* 37 (1): 103–120.

Marlatt, G. Alan. 1996. "Harm Reduction: Come as You Are." *Addictive Behaviors* 21 (6): 779–788.

Martin, Graham, Graime Currie, and Rachael Finn. 2009. "Reconfiguring or Reproducing Intra-professional Boundaries? Specialist Expertise, Generalist Knowledge and the 'Modernization' of the Medical Workforce." *Social Science and Medicine* 68:1191–1198.

Martinez, Alexis N., Ricky N. Bluthenthal, Jennifer Lorvick, Rachel Anderson, Neil Flynn, and Alex H. Kral. 2007. "The Impact of Legalizing Syringe Exchange

Programs on Arrests among Injection Drug Users in California." *Journal of Urban Health* 84 (3): 423–435.

Massachusetts Criminal Justice Training Council. 2000. *Controlled Substance Field Manual*. Randolph, MA: Massachusetts Criminal Justice Training Council.

Mattingly, Cheryl. 1998. "In Search of the Good: Narrative Reasoning in Clinical Practice." *Medical Anthropology Quarterly* 12 (3): 273–297.

———. 2006. "Pocahontas Goes to the Clinic: Popular Culture as Lingua Franca in a Cultural Borderland." *American Anthropologist* 108 (3): 494–501.

Matza, Tomas. 2009. "Moscow's Echo: Technologies of the Self, Publics, and Politics on the Russian Talk Show." *Cultural Anthropology* 24 (3): 489–522.

Mauer, Marc, and Meda Chesney-Lind, eds. 2002. *Invisible Punishment: The Collateral Consequences of Mass Imprisonment*. New York: New Press.

McKinney, Martha M., and Katherine M. Marconi. 2002. "Delivering HIV Services to Vulnerable Populations: A Review of Care Act–Funded Research." *Public Health Reports* 117 (2): 99–113.

MDPH (Massachusetts Department of Public Health). 2001. *HIV/AIDS Surveillance Report*. Boston: Massachusetts Department of Public Health HIV/AIDS Surveillance Unit.

———. 2010. *Who Is Currently Living with HIV/AIDS? March 2010*. Boston: Massachusetts Department of Public Health HIV/AIDS Surveillance Unit.

Meister, Joel, Louise Warrick, Jill de Zapién, and Anita Wood. 1992. "Using Lay Health Workers: Case Study of a Community-Based Prenatal Intervention." *Journal of Community Health* 17 (1): 37–51.

Melhuus, Marit. 1999. "Insisting on Culture?" *Social Anthropology* 7 (1): 65–80.

Mercer, Kobena. 1994. *Welcome to the Jungle: New Positions in Black Cultural Studies*. New York: Routledge.

Metcalfe, Andrew. 1993. "Living in a Clinic: The Power of Public Health Promotions." *Australian Journal of Anthropology* 4 (1): 31–44.

Michael, Reed. 1996. "Expert Power and Control in Late Modernity: An Empirical Review and Theoretical Synthesis." *Organization Studies* 17 (4): 573–597.

Middleton, DeWight. 2010. *The Challenge of Human Diversity*. Prospect Heights, IL: Waveland Press.

Miller, Chris, and Yusuf Ahmad. 1997. "Community Development at the Crossroads: A Way Forward." *Policy and Politics* 25 (3): 269–284.

Miller, Peter. 1995. "Production, Identity and Democracy." *Theory and Society* 24: 427–467.

———. 2001a. "A Critical Review of the Harm Minimization Ideology in Australia." *Critical Public Health* 11 (2): 167–178.

———. 2001b. "Governing by Numbers: Why Calculative Practices Matter." *Social Research* 68 (2): 379–396.

Minkler, Meredith. 1992. "Community Organizing among the Elderly Poor in the United States: A Case Study." *International Journal of Health Services* 22 (2): 303–316.

Minkler, Meredith, and Nina Wallerstein. 1997. "Improving Health through Community Organization and Community Building." In *Health Behavior and Health Education*, edited by K. Glanz, F. Marcus Lewis, and B. K. Rimer, 241–269. San Francisco: Jossey-Bass.

Montoya, Michael. 2007. "Bioethnic Conscription: Genes, Race and Mexicana/o Ethnicity in Diabetes Research." *Cultural Anthropology* 22 (1): 94–128.

Moore, David, and Suzanne Fraser. 2006. "Putting at Risk What We Know: Reflecting on the Drug-Using Subject in Harm Reduction and Its Political Implications." *Social Science and Medicine* 62 (12): 3035–3047.

Morgen, Sandra. 2002. *Into Our Own Hands: The Women's Health Movement in the United States, 1969–1990.* New Brunswick, NJ: Rutgers University Press.

Mugford, Stephen. 1993. "Message in a Toilet." *International Journal of Drug Policy* 4 (3): 135–145.

Naples, Nancy. 1997. "The 'New Consensus' on the Gendered 'Social Contract': The 1987–1988 U.S. Congressional Hearings on Welfare Reform." *Signs* 22 (4): 907–945.

Nathan, Richard P., and Thomas L. Gais. 1999. *Implementing the Personal Responsibility Act of 1996: A First Look.* New York: SUNY Rockefeller Institute of Government. Available at http://www.rockinst.org/pdf/federalism/1999–01-implementing_the_personal_responsibility_act_of_1996_a_first_look.pdf.

Navarro, Vicente, ed. 2004. *The Political and Social Contexts of Health.* Amityville, NY: Baywood.

Neaigus, Alan, Mingfang Zhao, V. Anna Gyarmathy, Linda Cisek, Samuel R. Friedman, and Robert C. Baxter. 2008. "Greater Drug Injecting Risk for HIV, HBV, and HCV Infection in a City Where Syringe Exchange and Pharmacy Syringe Distribution Are Illegal." *Journal of Urban Health* 85 (3): 309–322.

Nicholas, Stephen W., Betina Jean-Louis, Benjamin Ortiz, Mary Northridge, Katherine Shoemaker, Roger Vaughan, Michaela Rome, Geoffrey Canada, and Vincent Hutchinson. 2005. "Addressing the Childhood Asthma Crisis in Harlem: The Harlem Children's Zone Asthma Initiative." *American Journal of Public Health* 95 (2): 245–249.

Nichter, Mark. 2003. "Harm Reduction: A Core Concern for Medical Anthropology." In *Risk, Culture, and Health Inequality: Shifting Perceptions of Danger and Blame,* edited by B. Harthorn and L. Oaks, 13–34. Westport, CT: Praeger.

Ning, Ana M. 2005. "Games of Truth: Rethinking Conformity and Resistance in Narratives of Heroin Recovery." *Medical Anthropology* 24:349–382.

O'Hare, Patrick, Russell Newcombe, Alan Matthews, Ernst Buning, and Ernest Drucker. 1992. *The Reduction of Drug-Related Harm.* London: Routledge.

O'Malley, Patrick. 1999. "Governmentality and the Risk Society." *Economy and Society* 28:138–148.

Omi, Michael, and Howard Winant. 1989. *Racial Formation in the United States: From the 1960s to the 1980s.* New York: Routledge.

O'Neil, John, Jeffrey Reading, and Audrey Leader. 1998. "Changing the Relations of Surveillance: The Development of a Discourse of Resistance in Aboriginal Epidemiology." *Human Organization* 57 (2): 230–237.

Ong, Aihwa. 1995. "Making the Biopolitical Subject: Cambodian Immigrants, Refugee Medicine and Cultural Citizenship in California." *Social Science and Medicine* 40 (9): 1243–1257.

———. 2006. *Neoliberalism as Exception: Mutations in Citizenship and Sovereignty.* Durham, NC: Duke University Press.

Ong, Aihwa, and Stephen J. Collier, eds. 2005. *Global Assemblages: Technology, Politics, and Ethics as Anthropological Problems.* Malden, MA: Blackwell.

Oppenheimer, Gerald. 2001. "Paradigm Lost: Race, Ethnicity and the Search for a New Population Taxonomy." *American Journal of Public Health* 91 (7): 1049–1055.

Osborne, Thomas. 1997. "Of Health and Statecraft." In *Foucault, Health and Medicine,* edited by A. Petersen and R. Bunton, 173–188. London: Routledge.

Oudshoorn, Nelly, and Trevor Pinch, eds. 2003. *How Users Matter: The Co-construction of Users and Technology.* Cambridge, MA: MIT Press.

Park, Peter. 1993. "What Is Participatory Research? A Theoretical and Methodological Perspective." In *Voices of Change: Participatory Research in the United States and*

Canada, edited by P. P. Park, M. Brydon-Miller, B. Hall, and T. Jackson, 1–20. Westport, CT: Bergin and Garvey.

Parker, Edith A., A. J. Schulz, Barbara Israel, and R. Hollis. 1998. "Detroit's East Side Village Health Worker Partnership: Community-Based Lay Health Advisor Intervention in an Urban Area." *Health Education and Behavior* 25 (1): 24–45.

Peacock, Ben. 2008. "Sex, Drugs, and Statistics: Researchers and Researched in the Sciences of Urban Marginality." Ph.D. diss., Department of Anthropology, University of California, Berkeley.

Petersen, Alan R. 1997. "Risk, Governance and the New Public Health." In *Foucault, Health and Medicine*, edited by A. Petersen and R. Bunton, 189–206. London: Routledge.

Petersen, Alan R., and Deborah Lupton. 1996. *The New Public Health: Discourses, Knowledges, Strategies*. London: Sage.

Petryna, Adriana. 2002. *Life Exposed: Biological Citizens after Chernobyl*. Princeton, NJ: Princeton University Press.

Pigg, Stacy Leigh. 2001. "Languages of Sex and AIDS in Nepal: Notes on the Social Production of Commensurability." *Cultural Anthropology* 16 (4): 481–541.

Polgar, Steven. 1979. *Applied, Action, Radical, and Committed Anthropology*. The Hague, Netherlands: Mouton.

Polikoff, Nancy D. 2008. *Beyond (Straight and Gay) Marriage: Valuing All Families under the Law*. Boston: Beacon Press.

Pollock, Mica. 2005. *Colormute: Race Talk Dilemmas in an American School*. Princeton, NJ: Princeton University Press.

Poovey, Mary. 1995. *Making a Social Body: British Cultural Formations 1830–1864*. Chicago: University of Chicago Press.

Porter, Theodore. 1995. *Trust in Numbers: The Pursuit of Objectivity in Science and Public Life*. Princeton, NJ: Princeton University Press.

Power, Michael. 1994. "The Audit Society." In *Accounting as Social and Institutional Practice*, edited by A. G. Hopwood and P. Miller, 299–316. Cambridge: Cambridge University Press.

Prince, Russell, Robin Kearns, and David Craig. 2006. "Governmentality, Discourse and Space in the New Zealand Health Care System, 1991–2003." *Health and Place* 12 (3): 253–266.

Procacci, Giovanna. 1991. "Social Economy and the Government of Poverty." In *The Foucault Effect: Studies in Governmentality*, edited by G. Burchell, C. Gordon, and P. Miller, 151–168. Chicago: University of Chicago Press.

Rabinow, Paul. 1996. "Artificiality and Enlightenment: From Sociobiology to Biosociality." In *Essays on the Anthropology of Reason*, 91–111. Princeton, NJ: Princeton University Press.

———. 2005. "Midst Anthropology's Problems." In *Global Assemblages: Technology, Politics, and Ethics as Anthropological Problems*, edited by A. Ong and S. J. Collier, 40–53. Malden, MA: Blackwell.

Raco, Mike, Gavin Parker, and Joe Doak. 2006. "Reshaping Spaces of Local Governance? Community Strategies and the Modernisation of Local Government in England." *Environment and Planning C. Government and Policy* 4 (24): 475–496.

Rago, William V. 1996. "Struggles in Transformation: A Study in TQM, Leadership, and Organizational Culture in a Government Agency." *Public Administration Review* 56 (3): 227–234.

Rapp, Rayna. 1999. *Testing Women, Testing the Fetus: The Social Impact of Amnio-centesis in America*. New York: Routledge.

Reardon, Jenny. 2005. *Race to the Finish: Identity and Governance in an Age of Genomics*. Princeton, NJ: Princeton University Press.

Reed-Danahay, Deborah, and Caroline Brettell. 2008. *Citizenship, Political Engagement, and Belonging: Immigrants in Europe and the United States*. New Brunswick, NJ: Rutgers University Press.

Reeder, Leo. 1978. "The Patient-Client as Consumer." In *Dominant Issues in Medical Sociology*, edited by H. Schwartz and C. Kart, 111–117. Reading, MA: Addison-Wesley.

Reinarman, Craig, and Harry Levine, eds. 1997. *Crack in America: Demon Drugs and Social Justice*. Berkeley: University of California Press.

Riccio, James, and Yeheskel Hasenfeld. 1996. "Enforcing a Participation Mandate in a Welfare-to-Work Program." *Social Service Review* 70 (4): 516–541.

Riley, Diane, and Pat O'Hare. 2000. "Harm Reduction: History, Definition, and Practice." In *Harm Reduction: National and International Perspectives*, edited by J. A. Inciardi and L. D. Harrison, 1–26. Newbury Park, CA: Sage.

Robertson, Ann. 2001. "Biotechnology, Political Rationality and Discourses on Health Risk." *Health, Risk and Society* 5 (3): 293–310.

Robins, Steven. 2009. "Humanitarian Aid beyond 'Bare Survival': Social Movement Responses to Xenophobic Violence in South Africa." *American Ethnologist* 36 (4): 637–650.

Rock, Melanie. 2005. "Reconstituting Populations through Evidence-Based Medicine: An Ethnographic Account of Recommending Procedures for Diagnosing Type 2 Diabetes in Clinical Practice Guidelines." *Health (London)* 9 (2): 241–266.

Roe, Gordon. 2005. "Harm Reduction as Paradigm: Is Better Than Bad Good Enough? The Origins of Harm Reduction." *Critical Public Health* 15:243–250.

Rose, Nikolas. 1998. *Inventing Our Selves: Psychology, Power and Personhood*. Cambridge: Cambridge University Press.

———. 1999. *Powers of Freedom: Reframing Political Thought*. Cambridge: Cambridge University Press.

———. 2006. *The Politics of Life Itself: Biomedicine, Power, and Subjectivity in the Twenty-First Century*. Princeton, NJ: Princeton University Press.

Rose, Nikolas, and Carlos Novas. 2005. "Biological Citizenship." In *Global Assemblages: Technology, Politics, and Ethics as Anthropological Problems*, edited by A. Ong and S. J. Collier, 439–463. Malden, MA: Blackwell.

Rosenberg, Charles. 1987. *The Care of Strangers: The Rise of America's Hospital System*. Baltimore: Johns Hopkins University Press.

Rothschild, Debra. 1998. "Treating the Resistant Substance Abuser: Harm Reduction (Re)Emerges as Sound Clinical Practice." *In Session: Psychotherapy in Practice* 4 (1): 25–35.

Salber, Eva. 1979. "The Lay Advisor as a Community Health Resource." *Journal of Health Politics, Policy and Law* 3 (4): 469–478.

Santiago-Irizarry, Vilma. 2001. *Medicalizing Ethnicity: The Construction of Latino Identity in a Psychiatric Setting*. Ithaca, NY: Cornell University Press.

Sargent, Carolyn, and Stéphanie Larchanché. 2009. "The Construction of 'Cultural Difference' and Its Therapeutic Significance in Immigrant Mental Health Services in France." *Culture, Medicine and Psychiatry* 33 (1): 2–20.

Scally, Gabriel, and Liam J. Donaldson. 1998. "Clinical Governance and the Drive for Quality Improvement in the New NHS in England." *British Medical Journal* 317 (7150): 61–65.

Scheper-Hughes, Nancy, and Margaret Lock. 1987. "The Mindful Body: A Prolegomenon to Future Work in Medical Anthropology." *Medical Anthropology Quarterly* 1 (1): 6–41.

Schoenberg, N. E., K. A. Campbell, J. F. Garrity, L. B. Snider, and K. Main. 2001. "The Kentucky Homeplace Project: Family Health Care Advisers in Underserved Rural Communities." *Journal of Rural Health* 17 (3): 179–186.

Schoepf, Brooke G. 2001. "International AIDS Research in Anthropology: Taking a Critical Perspective on the AIDS Crisis." *Annual Review of Anthropology* 30: 335–361.

Schofield, Barry. 2002. "Partners in Power: Governing the Self-Sustaining Community." *Sociology* 36 (3): 663–683.

Schram, Sanford. 2000. *After Welfare: The Culture of Postindustrial Social Policy.* New York: New York University Press.

Scott, Ellen K., Andrew S. London, and Glenda Gross. 2007. "'I Try Not to Depend on Anyone but Me': Welfare-Reliant Women's Perspectives on Self-Sufficiency, Work, and Marriage." *Sociological Inquiry* 4 (77): 601–625.

Scott, James. 1998. *Seeing Like a State: How Certain Schemes to Improve the Human Condition Have Failed.* New Haven, CT: Yale University Press.

Sharma, Aradhana. 2008. *Logics of Empowerment: Development, Gender and Governance in Neoliberal India.* Minneapolis: University of Minnesota Press.

Shaw, Susan. 2001. "Dependency Transformed: The Making of Neoliberal Subjects in a Massachusetts Community Health Center." Ph.D. diss., Department of Anthropology, University of North Carolina, Chapel Hill.

———. 2005. "The Politics of Recognition in Culturally Appropriate Care." *Medical Anthropology Quarterly* 19 (3): 290–309.

———. 2006. "Public Citizens, Marginalized Communities: The Struggle for Syringe Exchange in Massachusetts." *Medical Anthropology* 25 (1): 31–64.

———. 2010. "The Logic of Identity and Resemblance in Culturally Appropriate Health Care." *Health* 14(5): 523–544.

Shore, Cris, and Susan Wright. 1997. *Anthropology of Policy: Critical Perspectives on Governance and Power.* London: Routledge.

Simon, Sherry. 1990. "Rites of Passage: Translation and its Intents." *Massachusetts Review* 31 (1–2): 96–110.

———. 1996. *Gender in Translation: Cultural Identity and the Politics of Transmission.* New York: Routledge.

Singer, M. 1993. "Knowledge for Use: Anthropology and Community-Centered Substance Abuse Research." *Social Science and Medicine* 37 (1): 15–25.

———. 1994a. "AIDS and the Health Crisis of the Urban Poor: The Perspective of Critical Medical Anthropology." *Social Science and Medicine* 39 (7): 931–948.

———. 1994b. "Community-Centered Praxis: Toward an Alternative Non-dominative Applied Anthropology." *Human Organization* 53 (4): 336–344.

———. 1999. "Why Do Puerto Rican Injection Drug Users Inject So Often?" *Anthropology and Medicine* 6 (1): 31–58.

———. 2002. "Toward the Use of Ethnography in Health Care Program Evaluation." In *The Applied Anthropology Reader,* edited by J. McDonald, 88–104. Boston: Allyn and Bacon.

———. 2004. "Why Is It Easier to Get Drugs Than Drug Treatment in the United States?" In *Unhealthy Health Policy: A Critical Anthropological Examination,* edited by A. Castro and M. Singer, 287–301. Walnut Creek, CA: AltaMira Press.

Singer, M., Zhongke Jia, Jean Schensul, Margaret Weeks, and J. Bryan Page. 1992. "AIDS and the IV Drug User: The Local Context in Prevention Efforts." *Medical Anthropology* 14:285–306.

Singer, M., N. Romero-Daza, M. Weeks, and P. Pelia. 1995. "Ethnography and the Evaluation of Needle Exchange in the Prevention of HIV Transmission." In *Qualitative Methods in Drug Abuse and HIV Risk,* edited by E. Lambert,

R. Ashery, and R. Needle, 231–257. Rockville, MD: NIDA Research Monograph Series.

Singer, M., T. Stopka, C. Siano, K. Springer, G. Barton, K. Khoshnood, A. Gorry de Puga, and R. Heimer. 2000. "The Social Geography of AIDS and Hepatitis Risk: Qualitative Approaches for Assessing Local Differences in Sterile-Syringe Access among Injection Drug Users." *American Journal of Public Health* 90 (7): 1049–1056.

Singer, M., Margaret Weeks, and David Himmelgreen. 1995. "Sale and Exchange of Syringes." *Journal of Acquired Immune Deficiency Syndromes and Human Retrovirology* 10:104–106.

Small, D. 2007. "Fools Rush in Where Angels Fear to Tread: Playing God with Vancouver's Supervised Injection Facility in the Political Borderland." *International Journal of Drug Policy* 18 (1): 18–26.

Small, D., A. Glickman, G. Rigter, and T. Walter. 2010. "The Washington Needle Depot: Fitting Healthcare to Injection Drug Users Rather Than Injection Drug Users to Healthcare: Moving from a Syringe Exchange to Syringe Distribution Model." *Harm Reduction Journal* 7 (1): 1–12.

Smith, Anna Marie. 2007. *Welfare Reform and Sexual Regulation*. Cambridge: Cambridge University Press.

Sondik, Edward, Jacqueline Wilson Lucas, Jennifer Madans, and Sandra Surber Smith. 2000. "Race/Ethnicity and the 2000 Census: Implications for Public Health." *American Journal of Public Health* 90 (11): 1709–1713.

Spielman, S. E., C. A. Golembeski, M. E. Northridge, R. D. Vaughan, R. Swaner, B. Jean-Louis, K. Shoemaker, et al. 2006. "Interdisciplinary Planning for Healthier Communities: Findings from the Harlem Children's Zone Asthma Initiative." *Journal of the American Planning Association* 72 (1): 100–109.

Starr, Paul. 1982. *The Social Transformation of American Medicine*. New York: Basic Books.

Stein, Arlene. 2010. "Sex, Truths, and Audiotape: Anonymity and the Ethics of Exposure in Public Ethnography." *Journal of Contemporary Ethnography* 39:554–568.

Stein, Jay M. 2000. "Doing Right and Making Money: Attracting Corporate Investment via Social Development-Creating Healthy Communities." *Economic Development Review* 17 (1): 36–40.

Steinecke, Ann, and Charles Terrell. 2010. "Progress for Whose Future? The Impact of the Flexner Report on Medical Education for Racial and Ethnic Minority Physicians in the United States." *Academic Medicine* 85 (2): 236–245.

Stopka, Tom, Merrill Singer, Claudia Santelices, and Julie Eiserman. 2003. "Public Health Interventionists, Penny Capitalists, or Sources of Risk? Assessing Street Syringe Sellers in Hartford, Connecticut." *Substance Use and Misuse* 38 (9): 1345–1377.

Storper, Michael. 2000. "Lived Effects of the Contemporary Economy: Globalization, Inequality, and Consumer Society." *Public Culture* 12 (2): 375–409.

Subramanian, Subu, Jarvis T. Chen, David H. Rehkopf, Pamela D. Waterman, and Nancy Krieger. 2005. "Racial Disparities in Context: A Multilevel Analysis of Neighborhood Variations in Poverty and Excess Mortality among Black Populations in Massachusetts." *American Journal of Public Health* 95 (2): 260–266.

Sullivan, Louis W., and Ilana Suez Mittman. 2010. "The State of Diversity in the Health Professions a Century after Flexner." *Academic Medicine* 85 (2): 246–253.

Takeuchi, David T., and Sue-Je L. Gage. 2003. "What to Do with Race? Changing Notions of Race in the Social Sciences." *Culture, Medicine and Psychiatry* 27 (4): 435–445.

Taussig, Karen-Sue, Deborah Heath, and Rayna Rapp. 2003. "Flexible Eugenics: Technologies of the Self in the Age of Genetics." In *Genetic Nature/Culture: Anthropology and Science Beyond the Two-Culture Divide*, edited by A. Goodman, D. Heath, and S. Lindee, 58–76. Berkeley: University of California Press.

Taylor, Janelle. 2003a. "Confronting 'Culture' in Medicine's 'Culture of No Culture.'" *Academic Medicine* 78 (6): 555–559.

———. 2003b. "The Story Catches You and You Fall Down: Tragedy, Ethnography, and 'Cultural Competence.'" *Medical Anthropology Quarterly* 17 (2): 159–181.

Thomas, James, Eugenia Eng, Michele Clark, Jadis Robinson, and Connie Blumenthal. 1998. "Lay Health Advisors: Sexually Transmitted Disease Prevention through Community Involvement." *American Journal of Public Health* 88 (8): 1252–1253.

Thomas, Stephen. 2001. "The Color Line: Race Matters in the Elimination of Health Disparities." *American Journal of Public Health* 91 (7): 1046–1047.

Thompson, Delamie, Ann Smith, Terry Hallom, and E. Paul Durrenberger. 1999. "Power, Rhetoric and Partnership: Primary Health Care and Pie in the Sky." *Human Organization* 58 (1): 94–104.

Tollman, S. M. 1994. "The Pholela Health Centre: The Origins of Community-Oriented Primary Health Care." *South African Medical Journal* 84 (10): 653–658.

Tough, Paul. 2004. "The Harlem Project." *New York Times Magazine*, June 20, 44.

Treichler, Paula. 1989. "AIDS, Homophobia and Biomedical Discourse: An Epidemic of Signification." In *AIDS: Cultural Analysis, Cultural Activism*, edited by D. C. Crimp, 31–70. Cambridge, MA: MIT Press.

Turner, Nicol, John L. McKnight, and John P. Kretzmann. 1999. *A Guide to Mapping and Mobilizing the Associations in Local Neighborhoods: A Community Building Workbook*. Chicago: ACTA.

U.S. Department of Health and Human Services. 2007. "National Standards on Culturally and Linguistically Appropriate Services (CLAS)." Office of Minority Health. Available at http://minorityhealth.hhs.gov/templates/browse.aspx?lvl=2&lvlID=15.

Valente, T. W., R. K. Foreman, B. Jungue, and D. Vlahov. 1998. "Satellite Exchange in the Baltimore Needle Exchange Program." *Public Health Reports* 113 (Suppl. 1): 90–96.

Valverde, Mariana. 1998. *Diseases of the Will: Alcohol and the Dilemmas of Freedom*. Cambridge: Cambridge University Press.

Varenne, Hervé. 1986. "Drop In Anytime: Community and Authenticity in American Everyday Life." In *Symbolizing America*, edited by H. Varenne, 209–228. Lincoln: University of Nebraska Press.

Wacquant, Loic. 1993. "Urban Outcasts: Stigma and Division in the Black American Ghetto and the French Urban Periphery." *International Journal of Urban and Regional Research* 17 (3): 366–383.

Wailoo, Keith. 2001. *Dying in the City of the Blues: Sickle Cell Anemia and the Politics of Race and Health*. Chapel Hill: University of North Carolina Press.

Waldby, Catherine. 1996. *AIDS and the Body Politic: Biomedicine and Sexual Difference*. London: Routledge.

Wallman, Katherine, Suzann Evinger, and Susan Schechter. 2000. "Measuring Our Nation's Diversity: Developing a Common Language for Data on Race/Ethnicity." *American Journal of Public Health* 90 (11): 1704–1708.

Walters, William. 1997. "The 'Active Society': New Designs for Social Policy." *Policy and Politics* 25 (3): 221–234.

Wellin, Edward. 1955. "Water Boiling in a Peruvian Town." In *Health, Culture and Community*, edited by Paul Benjamin, 71–103. New York: Russell Sage Foundation.

Weston, Kath. 1991. *Families We Choose: Lesbians, Gays, Kinship*. New York: Columbia University Press.

Willen, Sarah S., Antonio Bullon, and Mary-Jo DelVecchio Good. 2010. "'Opening up a Huge Can of Worms': Reflections on a 'Cultural Sensitivity' Course for Psychiatry Residents." *Harvard Review of Psychiatry* 18 (4): 247–253.

Willging, Cathleen E. 2005. "Power, Blame, and Accountability: Medicaid Managed Care for Mental Health Services in New Mexico." *Medical Anthropology Quarterly* 19 (1): 84–102.

Williams, Brackette. 1991. *Stains on My Name, War in My Veins: Guyana and the Politics of Cultural Struggle*. Durham, NC: Duke University Press.

———. 1995. "The Public I/Eye: Conducting Fieldwork to Do Homework on Homelessness and Begging in Two U.S. Cities." *Current Anthropology* 36 (1): 25–51.

Williams, Raymond. 1976. *Keywords*. New York: Oxford University Press.

Winant, Howard. 1994. *Racial Conditions: Politics, Theory, Comparisons*. Minneapolis: University of Minnesota Press.

Woolf, Steven, Robert Johnson, George Fryer, George Rust, and David Satcher. 2008. "The Health Impact of Resolving Racial Disparities: An Analysis." *American Journal of Public Health* 98 (Suppl. 1): S26–S28.

Wright, Kai. 2007. "The 'Colorblind' Attack on Your Health." *ColorLines*, March 1, 2007. Available at http://colorlines.com/archives/2007/03/the_colorblind_attack_on_your_health.html.

Wynne, Brian. 2001. "Creating Public Alienation: Expert Cultures of Risk and Ethics on GMOs." *Science as Culture* 10 (4): 445–482.

Young, Alicia L., and Sarah R. Wunsch. 2002. "*Commonwealth v. Maria Landry*, Defendant, Appellant: On a Report from the Lynn District Court. Appellant's Amended Brief, Addendum and Appendix." New York: American Civil Liberties Union Foundation of Massachusetts, April 24. Available at http://www.aclu.org/files/FilesPDFs/landry.pdf.

Index

Access to health care, 1, 12, 30, 126, 127, 188

Accountability, 24, 72–73, 80, 85, 130, 157

Addiction, 161, 163–164, 178n, representations of, 130–131

Advanced marginalization, 7, 31, 132

Advocacy, 30, 31, 105, 157, 167, 182, 184

Agencies, community-based, 34, 48, 49, 68, 81

Anderson, Joan, 123

Assemblage, 32, 34, 41, 45, 174, 181–182

Assets mapping, 57

Authenticity, 36, 38, 43–44, 45, 47. *See also* Community; Identity

Barker, Judith, 24n6

Benson, Peter, 122, 123

Biocitizenship, 29–30, 163–164, 182. *See also* Citizenship; Injection drug users (IDUs)

Biosociality, 19, 20, 29, 31

Bourdieu, Pierre, 59

Campbell, Nancy, 137n, 158n

Cant, Sarah, 115n7

Castel, Robert, 137

Citizenship, 182–183; and community health, 29, 58, 93, 186; and gender, 24; technologies of, 15, 35, 37, 40, 45, 63, 94

CLAS (culturally and linguistically appropriate services) standards, 38, 104, 106–107, 126–127. *See also* Cultural competence; Culturally appropriate health care (CAHC)

Class, 21

Cohn, Sandra, 79n7

Collier, Stephen, 124

Comaroff, John and Jean, 20, 25, 108, 115–116n8

Community, 3, 49, 117, 129, 186, 189; as assemblage, 45; capacity of, 94, 96–99, 189; and common needs, 59; as "hard to reach," 51, 52; and identity, 15, 38, 46, 48, 50, 52, 60, 117, 129, 186, 189; mapping of, 66–68; meanings of, 45, 47, 54, 55, 56, 59–60, 71, 102, 185, 187; organizer/organizing of, 44, 45, 56, 57, 58, 59, 67, 98–99, 182, 185; participation in, 65, 79, 99–100, 185, 186; urban, 97; uses of, 26. *See also* Authenticity; Expertise: community-based

Community health, 3, 5, 21, 36; as assemblage, 185, 188; and biosociality, 29–31;

Community health (*continued*)
  discourse of, 157; and governance 17, 18,
  20, 21, 66, 93, 185–187; and the medically underserved, 55; participation in,
  99; research on, 37; struggles over, 25,
  30, 184; urban, 21. *See also* Citizenship;
  Government/governance
Community Health Advocates (CHAs), 15,
  37, 103, 186; as agents of the state, 44,
  53–54, 100, 101; as community organizers, 70; identities of, 47–48, 50, 51, 92,
  93; pastoral role of, 53, 95; and Welfare-
  to-Work, 76–77, 87, 92
Community health centers, 38
Conscientization (Freire), 62. *See also*
  Education: as participatory
Consumer: of health care, 79, 80n; of social
  services, 73, 79, 80n, 95–96
Creed, Gerald, 20, 187
Crehan, Kate, 57, 58n
Cruikshank, Barbara, 34, 40
Cultural competence, 12, 109, 188; industry of, 16, 105. *See also* CLAS (culturally
  and linguistically appropriate services)
  standards; Culturally appropriate health
  care (CAHC); Education: and cultural
  competence; Education: cultural competence education as modularized knowledge
Culturally appropriate health care (CAHC),
  11, 16, 38, 103–105, 126; effectiveness
  of, 125; resistance to, 112–114; as standardized knowledge, 108, 116, 117, 123,
  128; technologies of, 23, 105–107, 110–
  112, 118, 120, 122, 124, 127. *See also*
  CLAS (culturally and linguistically appropriate services) standards; Cultural
  competence
Culture, 121, 124, 127

Davis, Mark, 146n
de la Cadena, Marisol, 25
Deleuze, Gilles, 174n
Dependency, 81n; and addiction, 133, 161;
  medicalization of, 85; welfare (character-
  istics of), 84
Difference, 186, 188, 189; cultural, 11, 15,
  16, 37, 117, 120–121, 126; problems of,
  11, 38, 104–105, 110
Disparities, health. *See* Health disparities
Donovan, Mark, 161n
Drug abuse, 16, 153, 159, 167, 178
Drug treatment, 143, 164, 181

Drug use, 16, 153, 159, 167, 178
Drug users, 151. *See also* Injection drug
  users (IDUs)

Education: and cultural competence, 113–
  114, 126; cultural competence education
  as modularized knowledge, 114-116,
  119n; as participatory, 45, 46, 47, 56–57,
  63
Empowerment, 15, 35, 56, 68, 95, 185,
  186; and consumerism, 73; and harm
  reduction, 130, 159; meaning of, 94, 96,
  101; as model of CHA program, 38, 39,
  57, 58, 67, 74, 99, 101
Engaged research, 8, 9, 189
Epidemiology, 137–139
Epstein, Steven, 23, 27
Ethics: of drug use, 130, 140–141, 143,
  145, 147; in health care, 109, 110, 117,
  118, 124; in research, 5–6, 8; and self-
  reflection, 112. *See also* Engaged research
Ethnicity: census categories for, 27; and
  community, 24–25, 38, 51, 54; and community health, 25; and governance, 26;
  meaning of, 15, 28; production of, 19–
  20, 117; representations of, 25–28, 139n
Ethnography: of drug use, 2, 137, 142,
  145–147, 148, 152, 153–155; and harm
  reduction norms, 139, 147; politics of, 5
Expertise, 107, 114–115, 122; ambivalence
  toward, 116, 118, 121, 123, 125; community-based, 52, 54, 91; cultural, 16, 23,
  104, 105, 107–108, 113, 115–116, 119,
  125–126, 128
Explanatory models, 122

Feldman, Allen, 7
Fraser, Nancy, 91
Freire, Paolo, 47, 57

Gastaldo, Denise, 99n27
Gender, 24, 57–59, 93, 95
Giddens, Anthony, 34
Gilroy, Paul, 28
Governing mentalities, 138; of drug use,
  133, 157–158; of harm reduction, 140;
  of risk, 137
Government/governance, 19, 20, 39, 130,
  156–157, 165; and community health,
  29, 131; ethics of, 35; and identity categories, 26–27, 151; modes of, 30, 34;
  neoliberal, 54, 55n, 82–83, 99, 127,
  186, 189; and risk, 138; techniques of,

94, 100–101, 131, 136, 157. *See also*
Citizenship: technologies of
Governmentality, 18, 32–35, 40, 41, 68,
130
Guattari, Felix, 174n
Gupta, Akhil, 40

Hacking, Ian, 138–139
Harm reduction, 16, 139–140, 158, 162,
176–177, 180, 182, 187, 189; discourse
on, 130, 140, 142; norms of, 135, 136,
144–145, 147, 148, 152, 153, 154, 157,
178
Harvey, David, 32, 33, 34, 55n
Health, social determinants of, 69, 127,
132, 136, 184
Health care reform, 188
Health disparities, 20, 26, 105, 127,
131–132, 184; discourse on, 19, 21–22,
28, 59, 188
Health education, radical, 9
Health promotion, 19
HIV, prevention of, 16, 31, 130, 131, 144,
173
Home visitors, 65
Horton, Sarah, 24n6
Humility, cultural, 119

Identity: and biopower, 29; categories of,
31, 56, 151; collective, 31, 157; emergence of, 30; ethnic, 28, 108. *See also*
Authenticity; Community
Injection drug users (IDUs), 16, 136, 138,
151, 161–162, 182; and biocitizenship,
30, 182; stigma surrounding, 132–133,
157, 158, 161, 180. *See also* Durg abuse;
Drug treatment

The Joint Commission, 107n5, 126
Joseph, Miranda, 20, 60, 93, 187

Kleinman, Arthur, 122, 123

Lakoff, Andrew, 124
Lay health advisors, 46, 64–65, 69. *See also*
Community Health Advocates (CHAs)
Li, Tania, 52n
Limoncelli, Stephanie, 83n11
Lovell, Anne, 79n7, 150
Lupton, Deborah, 84n14

Marinetto, Michael, 99n26
Matza, Tomas, 127n

Mead, Lawrence, 93
Meister, Joel, 51n6
Melhuus, Marit, 108
Metcalfe, Andrew, 99n25
Methadone, 141n
Minkler, Meredith, 47

Naples, Nancy, 84n15
Needle exchange. *See* Syringe exchange
Neoliberalism, 3, 15, 23–24, 80, 82–83,
97, 160; neoliberal state, 33, 79. *See also*
Government/governance
Ning, Ana, 141–142

Ong, Aihwa, 29
Oppression, 60
Outcome funding, 80
Outreach workers, 16, 51, 54n9, 64–65,
69, 132, 147, 186. *See also* Community
Health Advocates (CHAs); Lay health
advisors

Paraphernalia, criminal possession of, 153,
149n. *See also* Syringe exchange
Personal Responsibility and Work
Opportunity Reconciliation Act
(PRWORA), 78. *See also* Welfare-to-
Work
Policy, 24, 31, 35, 78, 83; and drugs, 153;
and HIV prevention, 181; and syringe
exchange, 156, 162; and welfare reform,
102
Political economy, 23–25, 123, 130
Pollock, Mica, 25n8
Population-based health, 64, 65–66, 68–70,
129, 130, 160, 179
Privilege, white, 31, 139n
Procacci, Giovanna, 81n9
Professionalization, 51
Public health, 21; as assemblage, 3; and
biopower, 31, 39
Public-private partnerships, 78

Quality Improvement (QI), 109, 110, 125

Racism, 115, 117, 118
Rationality, instrumental, 108, 122, 123
Reason, technological, 114, 117, 122,
123–124
Recognition, 20, 29, 31, 37, 105
Representation, 55, 56, 59
Research, engaged, 8, 9, 189
Resemblance and CHAs, 51

Responsibility, personal, 143; in harm reduction, 130, 147, 150, 154, 157, 159–160, 182, 188; in welfare policy 74. *See also* Self-sufficiency

Rhodes, Tim, 146n

Risk, 84n14, 130, 150, 166; categories of, 129, 136, 137, 138, 154, 189; discourse on, 138; "emic" categories of, 148–149, 152; information about, 129, 131, 148; and populations, 135, 137, 138; representations of, 136, 137, 148; risk behavior, 135; risk society, 137

Robins, Steven, 182

Rose, Nikolas, 3, 67, 83n10, 126, 174n

Ryan White Care Act, 161n

Schram, Sanford, 78–79, 84–85, 91

Scott, James, 56, 68, 154

Segregation, 25, 64

Self-sufficiency, 15, 35, 78, 83, 95, 96. *See also* Responsibility, personal

Sharma, Aradhana, 34, 40, 179

Sharma, Ursula, 115n7

Simon, Sherry, 61

Singer, Merrill, 130

Social movements, 59, 99, 118, 139, 154, 182, 184, 187, 188

Subjectivity, 60, 186, 189; of drug users, 158, 165, 175, 179; of health care providers, 108, 109, 121; of welfare recipients, 52, 92

Subject positions, 2, 5, 19, 21, 35, 56, 129, 131, 154, 185, 189

Substance abuse, 16, 153, 159, 167, 178

Syringe exchange, 14, 16–17, 130, 156, 166–167; and accountability, 168, 169–171, 183, 187; biopolitics of, 163–164, 166–167, 170, 175; and continuum of care, 157, 162, 165–166, 174, 179–181, 183; effectiveness of, 169; funding of, 160, 162n; legal status of, 168, 171–172; secondary exchange, 169

Thompson, Delamie, 50n

Translation, linguistic, 61–62; conceptual, in education, 62–63

Universal precautions, 116

Wailoo, Keith, 64

Wallerstein, Nina, 47

War on Drugs, 143, 147

Welfare assistance, 78, 81n

Welfare reform, 83; and contracts, 79, 90. *See also* Welfare-to-Work

Welfare-to-Work, 15, 73; case managers, 72, 82, 91; eligibility requirements, 75–77, 86–87, 102; enrollment, 87; funding flowchart, 74; and governance, 101; and job training, 75, 89, 90–91, 92; participation in, 72, 99–100; program implementation, 76–77, 82; and work experience, 83, 88–90

Winant, Howard, 28

Woolf, Steven, 22n2

Susan J. Shaw is Associate Professor in the School of Anthropology at the University of Arizona.